AF266740

TAKING CHARGE

OF YOUR BODY

MANAGING YOUR MUSCLES, BONE, AND CONNECTIVE TISSUE HEALTH

Richard L. Van Buskirk, DO, PhD

Author's Tranquility Press
ATLANTA, GEORGIA

Copyright © 2024 by Richard L. Van Buskirk, DO, PhD

All rights reserved. No part of this publication may be reproduced, distributed or transmitted in any form or by any means, including photocopying, recording, or other electronic or mechanical methods, without the prior written permission of the publisher, except in the case of brief quotations embodied in critical reviews and certain other noncommercial uses permitted by copyright law. For permission requests, write to the publisher, addressed "Attention: Permissions Coordinator," at the address below.

Richard L. Van Buskirk, DO, PhD/Author's Tranquility Press
3900 N Commerce Dr. Suite 300 #1255
Atlanta, GA 30344
www.authorstranquilitypress.com

Ordering Information:
Quantity sales. Special discounts are available on quantity purchases by corporations, associations, and others. For details, contact the "Special Sales Department" at the address above.

Taking Charge of your Body:
Managing and Healing your Musculoskeletal Body/Richard L. Van Buskirk, DO, PhD

Hardback: 978-1-965463-51-2
Paperback: 978-1-965463-23-9
eBook: 978-1-965463-24-6

Table of Contents

Dedication

This book is dedicated to Robert Dzmura, DO, a wonderful, knowledgeable and humble Healer who taught me how to be a physician in the truest sense of the word. It is also dedicated to all of my patients who have been endlessly patient with me over the years. I wish to thank my wife, Monica Van Buskirk who believed in this project and helped me get it published. I also wish to thank Gayle Guynup whose editorial skill kept the language of this book from being too academic and James Flynn who provided the photographs that translate words into actions you can copy.

Richard Van Buskirk, DO, PhD
Sarasota, Florida
Fall 2024

INTRODUCTION

You say that you have pain because something is not right in your bones, joints, muscles, tendons or nerves. What do you do about it? What is the cause? How do you prevent it? When you already have a problem with your muscles, tendons or joints what can you do about it? What does all that medical terminology the doctor uses to explain things really mean? Why did a simple stumble result in pain no different than if you had fallen? When you stand or sit why do you look crooked? How do you manage your muscular and skeletal body?

In my thirty plus years of medical practice these and many similar questions have been asked over and over again. As I answered my patients they frequently asked where these answers are written down. This book is written to give you those answers. If you are trying to deal with these kinds of problems this book is for you. Understanding your body and knowing what to do when things are not working well is the goal of this book.

My medical practice focuses on what is termed neuromusculoskeletal medicine. I specialize in diagnosing and medically managing problems that have developed in patients' necks, backs, arms, legs, hips and even their heads. I practice orthopedics without resorting to surgery. In fact, part of my focus is helping people avoid surgery.

This book has developed and evolved over many years. After many starts and stops, I am most thankful it has come together with the help of my wife, Monica Van Buskirk and my editor, Gayle Guynup. I also want to thank James Flynn for his expert photography.

This book is not a medical manual. It is intended to be a reference to help you understand, make informed decisions about and maintain your body. It is not a substitute for proper evaluation and treatment by your doctor. It is not intended to substitute for proper treatment by a licensed physical or occupational therapist.

I hope this book is helpful.

Richard Van Buskirk, DO, PhD

CHAPTER 1
Life is Movement

The focus in this book is to understand, correct and maintain the balance and useability of those parts of the physical body that allow us to act and interact in the world: the muscles, tendons, ligaments, bone and fascia and the brain, spinal cord and nerves that manage them. Together the muscles, tendons, bones and fascia are termed in medicine and biology the musculoskeletal system. The brain, spinal cord and muscles are termed the nervous system.

We operate in and on the world using our muscles, tendons, joints, ligaments and bones. We use them for everything we do. Walking, standing, sitting, running, jumping, watching a movie, writing a book and playing a game all require this complex system of bone, muscles and tendons. When the musculoskeletal system is working well, we tend to take it for granted. When it isn't working well, we are very aware of the limitations and often pain. This book is written to help us understand this complex system: how it works, what happens when things go wrong and what we can do to help correct problems when they arise.

I remember standing in a small exam room with my medical mentor and one of his patients as he told the patient, "You must start moving. Life is movement. If you don't move, you're dead." As a medical intern I thought the speech was effective but a bit exaggerated. Now, almost 30 years later, I'm convinced Dr. Dzmura was absolutely right.

This book is about moving our bodies. It is not about a prescribed series of exercises. Rather it is written to help you understand your body, how its muscles, tendons, ligaments, joints, bones and nervous system work together. Because the term "musculoskeletal" is uncommon in everyday use and does not easily role off the tongue, I choose to use the term "soma" in this book to refer to this complex system. In both ancient Greek and Japanese, the term soma means body. Medically we sometimes use the term soma to mean all parts of the physical body except the reproductive cells. However, because each of the other systems in the body have their own terms (like heart, cardiac, brain and nervous system)

I will use *soma* to be that part of the body that includes the muscles, connective tissue and bones. When used as an adjective to modify another word the term will be "somatic." Thus, pain in the body would be somatic pain. As we will see throughout this book, all somatic parts including muscles, tendons, ligaments, bones, joints and fascia are interdependent and act in partnership with the nervous system to produce a dynamic, balanced and healthy living being. A major purpose of this book is to help us understand how these elements operate normally.

This book is also about common things that happen to our soma and what can go wrong. It is about events that can limit our ability to move and function. It is sometimes about pain. This book also includes methods you can use to correct the failures and partial failures that seem to build up over time. It is also about how to prevent them. Above all, it is about healing our somatic body and how we can restore that strong dynamic balance that allows us to move. It is about life.

What can you do when you develop pain or stiffness and restriction somewhere in your body? What does it mean? Why is it there? Above all, how do you make it go away and stay away? Most of us will need to search for answers to these questions at least once in our lives. If we fall or are injured, these questions and their answers can become quite important.

As a medical physician dealing with the nervous system and the soma and their interactions, I get these questions all the time. All too often patients who come to me have been to many other physicians and non-physicians who deal with the soma looking for answers. In significant part the purpose of this book is to provide the kinds of answers that I had to learn and then teach my patients over the years.

In my many years of practice I have had people see me for a wide variety of medical problems. But for the past 15 years most have come to my practice because of some problem related to pain or restriction involving their soma. Pain is poorly understood even though most of us will experience it many times in our lives. Part of the purpose of this book is to help us understand what is going on when we have pain. The assumption behind this book is that pain is primarily an effect or a warning sign. Understanding its meaning in a particular case may well hold the solution to the problem.

Not too long ago a new patient came to see me. He said that he had been everywhere with the pain in his neck. His neck pain had come on seemingly overnight about two months before. He had done nothing to injure it. After a few days when his neck pain didn't go away, he went to see his primary care physician. His primary care physician told him that it was nothing and would go away over time. He suggested the patient ice his neck, told him to take a couple of Ibuprofen, and gave him prescriptions for a muscle relaxer. The man then went to his massage therapist. The massage therapist told him the muscles were rock hard and needed to be stretched and released. This helped for a few hours and then his pain came back. On the advice of a friend, he went to see a chiropractor. Years before he had seen another chiropractor who had helped him with an episode of low back pain, but that chiropractor had retired. The new chiropractor took X-rays and told him that his neck had arthritis and would need to be adjusted three times a week. After two adjustments his neck pain was worse and he decided not to go back. In fact, his pain was bad enough that he went to the Emergency Room where he was seen by a Physician's Assistant. The PA ordered an MRI of his neck. The ER doctor examined the MRI and told him he had a small disc herniation which was later properly diagnosed as disc degeneration, and some arthritis. He gave him an injection of Demerol, a narcotic, and sent him home on another muscle relaxant and a prescription for yet another narcotic, Hydrocodone. He also instructed him to follow up with a neurosurgeon. When he saw the neurosurgeon, he was told that there really wasn't anything that should be treated surgically. He was referred for four weeks of physical therapy. After three weeks of physical therapy and very little progress he came to see me on the advice of another friend.

As I examined him, I discovered that his left second toe had a blackened nail, indicating that it had been injured sometime in the not-too-distant past. When I asked him about the toe he was surprised and confused. He didn't see any connection between a blackened toenail and his neck pain. I explained to him that I was looking at him as a whole person. The strategy of looking only at his neck had not yielded satisfactory results so maybe the next step was to look at his whole body. The arthritis and disc degeneration in his neck had undoubtedly been there long before he developed pain. The solution was to look elsewhere.

Returning to the question of his foot, the patient recalled that he had hit his foot and stumbled badly around the time his neck pain started. In fact, he was pretty sure he had broken his toe. He knew that there was little to do for a broken toe except to tape it to the neighboring toe. In his interaction with the doctor and others he didn't say anything about it. As we discussed what had happened, he said he limped for a while after the toe injury though that had improved. He also volunteered that over-all he was much stiffer than before the injury. The stiffness included his low back, hips and legs as well as his neck. He expressed some surprise that after the initial pain in his toe, the only thing that hurt him was his neck.

As with most of my patients this became a teaching moment. I always try to explain what is going on. My work is never complete unless the patient walks out with a better understanding of their body and how it works.

The patient's story and symptoms are key parts of finding out what's going on. However, in the end, I always turn to the evaluation of the patient's body, focusing primarily on the muscles, tendons, ligaments, bones, joints and nerves. In this patient's case I found a pattern of restrictions involving not only his neck but his upper and lower back, hips and legs. Treating only the restrictions present in his neck would have been unsuccessful, as they had been for others who tried to treat him. The cause of his neck pain was in the whole-body pattern of restriction that developed from stumbling and injuring his toe.

As I treated the pattern of somatic imbalances that had grown from his simple stumble and toe injury the patient felt the pain in his neck shift and begin to release even before I began treating his neck. His surprise and relief were evident as he experienced the truth of the idea that both the injury and the treatment involved the whole body.

After the treatment was complete, he stood up with little pain or restriction. My final job was to discuss with him what he needed to do afterward: drink lots of water, rest for a day and take an anti-inflammatory of choice. After that he needed to do some stretches and start (in his case restart) his exercise program.

OSTEOPATHY

I am an osteopathic physician (DO) who specializes in problems involving the muscles, bones, joints and nervous system. I am not what is commonly referred to as a "pain doctor" or pain management specialist. I examine and treat people who have abnormal function, pain and restriction in their muscles, tendons, ligaments, bones and joints throughout the body. In medical terms, I treat the musculoskeletal system. As noted earlier, use of the term "musculoskeletal" is awkward. However quite literally no other term exists in English that describes the complex system of nerves, muscles, tendons, joints and bones that are the largest component of our body by weight and volume. That is the reason I have chosen to use the term "soma" to indicate the musculoskeletal system.

The osteopathic medical profession developed in the American Midwest more than 125 years ago. It was founded by an M.D., Andrew Taylor Still, who had serious reservations about the medicine of his day. Because his ideas and methods were not accepted by the medical doctors of the day, Dr. Still opened the first osteopathic medical school in Kirksville, Missouri in 1892. Its graduating physicians were given the title Doctor of Osteopathy or DO.

From the beginning, the osteopathic emphasis was on providing forms of treatment that would allow the body to heal itself. The physician was not the source of healing. The patient was. Osteopathic medicine was developed at a time when most of the available medicines were quite toxic, addicting or ineffective. In contrast, the osteopathic tradition emphasized use of manual interventions, lifestyle modifications and, when necessary, surgery to help the body heal itself.

The original osteopathic concept included the idea that removing restrictions in the body should result in disease improvement. All the other organs are embedded within the musculoskeletal system. Most of the functions of the other organs are as reliant on the integrity of this system as the body is on them. It made a great deal of sense to these early osteopathic physicians that improving muscle, bone and joint function could influence improvement of problems in other organs. According to the many books and journal articles published by the early osteopathic physicians, removing somatic restrictions did prove to be remarkably successful in improving disease. In fact, from the data available, the chance of surviving influenza during the 1918 influenza epidemic was better for a patient of an osteopathic physician than for one treated by an M.D.

The idea that manual interventions could help the body heal itself is not unique to the osteopathic profession. It is documented to go back to early Greek medicine. It is also a part of many other medical traditions worldwide including traditional Chinese and Japanese medicine, Ayurvedic medicine and some of the Native American medical traditions. In the United States, chiropractic developed at about the same time as osteopathic medicine and in the same part of the country.

What made the osteopaths unique among those following this line of thought was a strong western medical orientation. Osteopathic diagnosis followed the same logic and methods as those practiced by other medical doctors (M.D.s). Those medical problems that failed conservative treatment might end up in surgery just as it would in the medical system. Although early osteopathic physicians were often considered quacks by their M.D. colleagues, that, too, began to change by the 1940s. By that time osteopathic medical training was very similar to that of MDs, including the use of medications. However, it would be another 30 years before osteopathic physicians were granted equal practice rights with M.D.s in all parts of the country.

Today many osteopathic physicians are indistinguishable from their M.D. colleagues except for the slight difference in their perspective and their unique emphasis during training on the somatic aspects of diagnosis and treatment of disease. Modern osteopathic medicine still emphasizes the concept that it is the individual's whole body that does the healing. The physician can help provide a context in which good healing can occur. But the doctor does not heal the patient. Further, osteopathic physicians tend to look at the whole person rather than parts of the person.

It is true that many thoughtful physicians, whether M.D. or D.O., tend to look at both disease and health in a more "holistic" fashion today. However, many of the medical advances of the 20th century came by focusing on individual organs and their function in health and disease. An inevitable result was to split up medical care along lines defined by different organs and functions. That has led to the useful fiction that we can diagnose and treat diseased organs or systems with little regard for what the disease and treatment does to other systems. Because the original osteopathic model emphasized the interrelationship of all parts of the body, osteopathic physicians have tended to shy away from strictly organ-focused diagnosis and treatment.

The osteopathic profession emphasized the use of the muscles, bones, joints and nerve systems in the diagnosis and treatment of disease for much of its history. With the successes brought on by newer developments in diagnostic tests, medications and surgery, many osteopathic physicians now use much less of the original manual treatment. However, there are still those of us who include a strong emphasis on whole-body diagnosis and treatment including manual medicine.

HOW I FUNCTION AS A PHYSICIAN

When I look at a patient who comes to me with pain or inability to use a part of their body properly, I try to emphasize several points that will be covered in more detail later. First, as I see it, my job is to help their body help itself. I will not be doing the healing. The patient will. Second, all too often the pain they are experiencing may be the result of events at sites different from where they are experiencing pain. Third, their pain and restriction does not come from a failure to heal. If the injury was more than a month in the past, most of the time they have already healed. They just healed wrong. My job is to restart the healing process by helping the body to regain its proper balance. As it regains its balance this reinforces its memory of what constitutes normal function and balance. Fourth, what we will be doing is a process. In essence we are reeducating the body. Often the process takes time, particularly if the original injury was a long time in the past. Finally, the process of regaining normal healthy use of the muscles, joints, bones and nerves is not passive. It is not merely what I do as a physician that will help a person heal properly. What the patient does and does not do will play significant roles in how well he or she heals.

My specialty tends to cross a lot of lines that are often drawn between medical specialists: orthopedic surgeon, neurologist, rheumatologist, pain management doctor (anesthesiologists), and rehabilitation physicians (physiatrists). Some orthopedic surgeons who no longer perform surgeries practice a form of "orthopedic medicine" that is similar to what I practice. So do some physiatrists. However, because my practice includes manipulating the muscles, tendons, ligaments, joints, bones and nervous system I am a specialist rarely seen in American M.D. medicine, the manual medicine specialist. Coming out of the tradition of osteopathic medicine, I include somatic manipulation as an integral part of my medical diagnosis and treatment. It should be noted that outside of North America manual medicine is more frequently included in the M.D. medical toolbox.

There are many forms of manipulation of the muscles, joints, bones and nervous system that have been developed by the osteopathic profession. Most are gentle and do not cause much, if any, pain as they are applied. In the osteopathic tradition they are only applied after a careful detailed examination of the ease and restriction at multiple points throughout the body including, but not limited to, the area(s) of pain. If you come to me with a pain in your neck, I will evaluate your whole body. I will also look at your heart, lungs, and nervous system. I will look at your posture and how you move. I will listen carefully to your history and look at any diagnostic studies you have already had including labs and X-rays. I will include a detailed evaluation using my hands of the tissue texture, and movement of the rest of the spine, ribs, arms, hips, legs and muscles. Only when I know what is normal and what is not will I address somatic restrictions using manual medical methods.

Frequently my treatment includes a prescription for various forms of exercise and stretching to help patients deal with specific problems. I also prescribe medications as necessary for the control of pain or for dealing with muscle spasms. If the source of the problem is autoimmune arthritis, I may prescribe a disease-modifying medication. I also may give injections, particularly into joints, tendons, and bursa if nothing else helps. I might also inject with nerve blocking agents if necessary. I will include advice about any medications the patient might already be using that might affect their somatic systems. I will initiate diagnosis of any other disease processes that might be causing limitations of the function of the soma and nervous system dysfunction or contributing to their pain. I may send the patient back to their other physicians if their treatment for non-somatic problems needs modification. I will also include advice on those lifestyle changes I believe might benefit my patient.

Sometimes my advice will be to go ahead with a surgical procedure if that is the only viable option. However, most of the time I try to help people avoid surgery or the use of addictive drugs. For the most part my advice is not aimed at helping people who have had recent surgery and its attendant post-operative pain. However, understanding how and why it occurs may help us tolerate this kind of acute pain. Also, if the surgery is more than a couple weeks in the past and there is still restriction, dysfunction or pain, I will often become involved in trying to help the person recover.

FOCUSING ON THE MUSCULOSKELETAL BODY

This book is not focused on dysfunction and pain that comes from our internal organs. However, in a number of cases internal organ dysfunction has significant impact on the functioning of the rest of the body. Obviously, a stroke or a tumor in the brain could have a significant effect on how well we can use our muscles, tendons and joints. Similarly, heart disease and circulation problems, diabetes and thyroid disease will have major effects on function of the soma. The advice found in this book is based on an understanding that the soma does not exist in isolation. Part of this book is to help people understand how other organs have an impact on our soma. We will also explore what we can do to rebalance the soma in face of disease in other parts of the body.

A major purpose of this book is to help those who are having problems with their muscles, tendons, ligaments, joints and bones. Whether there is debilitating pain, mild pain, mere restriction or even the possibility of future pain, they need better answers. To know what is going on, how to treat it now and how to prevent problems in the future can be very useful. The purpose is to help people help themselves. Over the years I have provided many of my patients with self-help advice. Often the response has been to ask me where this advice has been written down. Many of them remembered the gist of what I told them. However, the details might have gone missing. To be honest most of this material hasn't been written down until now.

The other reason for this book is to explain to sufferers with musculoskeletal dysfunction and pain what is going on. Too often physicians don't do a very good job of explaining medical conditions in everyday language. Frequently patients look to other sources to try to understand what is happening. Sometimes those other sources aren't very reliable. I hope this book will help you understand better how the nervous system, bones, joints muscles and nerves work and what is happening when things go wrong and we develop restriction and pain.

The problem of body dysfunction is terribly common, particularly as we age. I have come to realize that not only do my patients need this material, but so do many others. So many people need advice. They want to understand why they can't move the way they used to. They are having pain and they want to know why. Even more, they need advice on how to get out of pain or at least to manage it. Many of the options commonly presented by modern medicine for managing muscle, tendon, joint and bone dysfunction and pain involve referrals to physical therapy, surgery and/or narcotics. This book provides advice for those who want other options. Hopefully all who are suffering from somatic dysfunction and pain will find this book useful.

CHAPTER 2
Normal Somatic Structure and Function

Understanding the mechanisms that allow us to move and operate in our world is a key to managing our bodies. Biomedical science has developed an almost molecular picture of these processes. Fortunately, we don't need to go deep into the woods in order to get the basic picture. We will be taking a step into them however, so please bear with me. You will benefit from this knowledge. Hopefully you will have at least a few "ah hah" moments as you read on.

Movement requires two things. There are the elements that cause the movement and there must be an architecture against which the moving element can operate. The architectural elements that the muscle cells operate on are the bones and connective tissues. The primary "mover" in our body is the contractile cell, otherwise known as a muscle cell. In a body like ours, made up of many cells, there also must be a coordinator of all this movement. That coordinator is our nervous system.

THE FASCIAL CONNECTION

The connective tissues are literally the skeleton of our soft tissues, the framework of our bodies. Another term for connective tissue is fascia (pronounced "fasha"). When massage therapists talk about a deep tissue or "myofascial" massage they are referring to a massage that stretches and relaxes our connective tissues (fascia) and muscles (myo).

Fascia defines, connects and supports all of our organs. Fascia consists of complex webs of protein fibers. Fascia can be loose or dense. It can be in the form of loose webs, sheets, multi-layered sheets, thick bundles and cables. Fascia wraps around every organ, defines the inner structure of each organ, defines the architectural relationships between organs and even defines the structure of our skin. Every cell in the body is supported in fascia. Clear to white in color, fascia is literally the matrix of our bodies. If we could remove all cellular elements of the body the fascia and our bones would be a ghost of our body: filmy, pale but recognizably human.

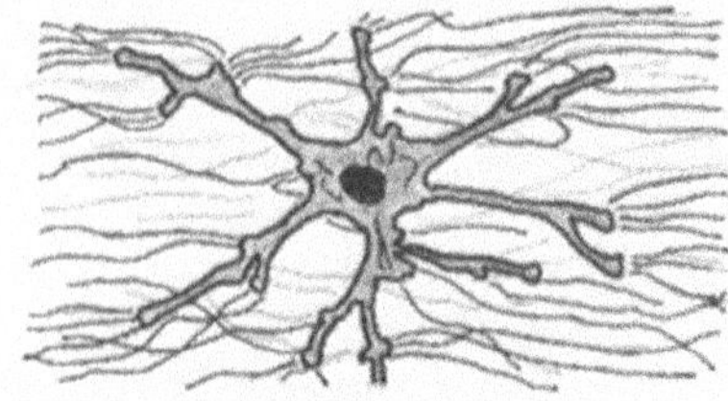

Fig. 2-1: A fibroblast and the protein fibers it produced.

Scattered through the fascia are the cells that produce and support the protein fibers (Fig. 2-1). These cells are called *fibroblasts*. The two primary connective tissue fiber types are *collagen* and *elastin*. Within the complex matrix of fibers, body fluid circulates, moving from arteries to veins and lymphatic channels. The fibers and fluid together support the fibroblasts, and any other cells embedded within the fascia matrix. Depending on the types of *collagen* fibers and the ratio of collagen to elastin, connective tissue has many different presentations in the body ranging from tendons and ligaments, to skin, cartilage, bone, blood vessels, internal structure for organs, and discs between the vertebrae.

FASCIA ALIVE

Most of us, if we think about fascia at all, think of it as unchanging, static. In reality, fascia is alive and dynamic. In addition to moving as the organs embedded within move, it also moves as our body moves. As a living tissue, cells in the fascia die and are replaced by new cells. This includes the fibroblasts. The dead cells are broken down and their waste is transferred to the bathing fluid where it moves into the veins and lymphatics. Protein doesn't last forever. It, too, degenerates and is then replaced by new protein. The collagen and elastin fibers are continuously being replaced.

This process of perpetual renewal keeps fascia healthy and prevents degradation. It allows for laying down new fibers along the lines of stress. Finally, it provides a healthy matrix in which the many different types of cells that make up our organs can thrive.

SOMATIC FASCIA

Frequently fascia is laid down in thick bands, cables and sheets. The tendons that connect a muscle to bone are one form of fascia. The thicker bands of tissue that surround a muscle are another form of fascia. Ligaments and joint capsules are also fascia.

In tendons, most fibers are collagen but are interspersed with elastin fibers that give tendons their flexibility and spring. Under a microscope, normal tendon fibers align parallel to the direction of stress (fig. 2-2a). That line of stress would be between the body of the muscle and the attachment of the tendon to bone. Repetitive stress along the axis of the tendon causes the parallel arrangement of the fibers, keeping them properly aligned.

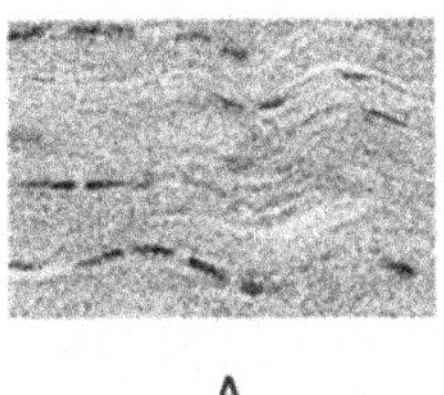

A

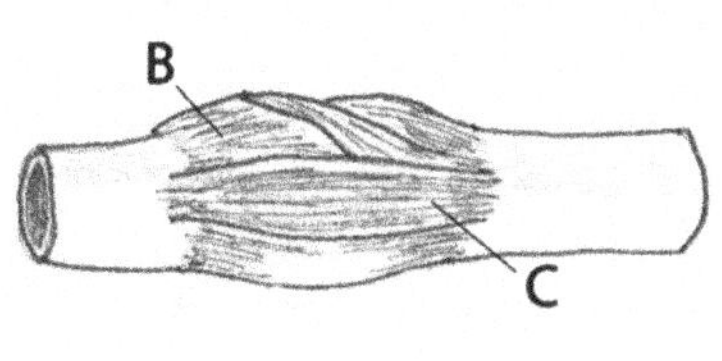

Fig. 2-2
A: tendon fibers aligned along the line of stress;
B: joint capsule;
C: ligament crossing the joint outside the joint capsule.

The joint between two bones is enclosed by connective tissue that binds the two bones together (Fig. 2-2b). The joint capsule encloses the joint and is organized in bands and sheets of parallel fibers that follow the lines of stress necessary to hold the joint together, while still allowing movement of one bone relative to the other. There may be many different bands with different orientations around the joint, but together they are arranged in a way to maintain the joint through its normal range of motion. The joint capsule is tight enough to keep fluid within the joint from leaking into the surrounding tissues.

Ligaments, meanwhile, are thick, tough bands of connective tissue that cross from one bone to another, inside or outside of the joint capsule (Fig. 2-2c). Unlike muscles, they have no embedded muscle cells. Ligaments act to limit the motion between two bones. Like tendons, the fibers in ligaments are typically laid out parallel to each other. They are quite resistant to force along the length of the ligament, but not as resistant to forces approaching from other angles.

BONES

Bone is a specialized form of connective tissue that provides the struts that allow us to stand or sit and operate in gravity. It differs from fascia because there are additional cells that specialize in laying down and maintaining calcium in the fiber matrix. Without bone we would be reduced to the structural equivalent of a jellyfish. The bone-building cells that lay down calcium in the fiber matrix are called *osteoblasts*. There is also another type of cell in the bone matrix called the *osteoclast* that is responsible for removing calcium. Together these two cell types continually remodel living bone. Like dense fascia, the bone matrix is laid down following the lines of force. For instance, in long bones the lines of force run along the length of the bone.

In dead bones, flexibility has been lost as the cells die and the fibrous matrix degenerates. Dead bone is like a rock made of calcium. It has no flexibility and no ability to remodel and regenerate. That is not the way living bone works. Living bone flexes or gives with increased force. When we walk or even more when we run or jump, the long bones of the leg flex a little, functioning like a spring.

Most bones have high density on the outside, while the inner core is more like a loose fibrous matrix with some thin bone dividers. Within this matrix is the birthplace of blood cells and a major source of stem cells, called bone marrow.

A FEW WORDS ABOUT OSTEOPOROSIS

While we are discussing bone let's take a moment to look at a very common disease of the bone, *osteoporosis*. When a person has osteoporosis, the bone osteoclasts are more active than the osteoblasts. The destruction exceeds the building of bone. Slowly the calcium leaches away, decreasing the strength of the bone. This makes the bone more likely to break at stress points. In its earliest stage, the weakening bone condition is termed *osteopenia*. As it progresses and the risk of fracture increases, it is called osteoporosis. Weight-bearing exercise and supplementation with at least 1200 mg of elemental calcium are very important in the prevention and treatment of osteoporosis. To allow the calcium to transfer from the gut into the bloodstream we also need vitamin D3. Although the body can make vitamin D3 in response to sunlight on the skin, we generally do not get enough sun exposure to produce an adequate amount of D3. Therefore, taking an oral supplement of D3 (at least 800 IU per day) is strongly recommended.

The standard medical treatment for osteoporosis is to use a type of medication called a *bisphosphonate*. These medications include Fosamax (*alendronate*), Actonel (*risedronate*), Boniva (*ibandronate*), and Reclast (*zoledronic acid*). These medications partially block the activity of the osteoclasts. Although this reverses the process by making the destructive process slower than the building process, the bone that is built is not exactly normal. The matrix looks different under the microscope. The new bone is stronger than it was, but without the flexibility that the bone originally had. After five years of bisphosphonate treatment, the long bones develop the possibility of breaking in the long shaft although such fractures remain uncommon. Another problem that can develop with bisphosphonates is a decreased resistance to bacterial infection around the teeth leading to bone death or osteonecrosis. Again, this is an uncommon problem.

Other medications used in the treatment of osteoporosis are based on the natural processes underlying the development and maintenance of bone. One, Forteo (*teriparatide*), mimics the naturally occurring parathyroid hormone PTH. PTH is responsible for the balance of the processes of breaking down and building up bone by causing the binding and release of calcium from bone. Interestingly, if the PTH levels are too high, the balance between the destructive and building processes fails with the destructive process winning. This is what happens when a parathyroid tumor develops in the area of the thyroid. The rapid destruction of bone leads to excessively high levels of calcium in the blood and causes muscle spasms, pain, racing heart and mental confusion.

The female hormone estrogen plays a significant role in the development of bone in girls as they go through puberty. With estrogen, most of the bone in adult women is maintained with normal strength, flexibility and density during a woman's reproductive years. Loss of estrogen is one of the primary reasons for the development of osteoporosis in women. Thus, estrogen supplementation can be used to help maintain stronger bones in women after menopause. However, other issues relating to the side effects of estrogen supplementation (hormone replacement therapy) after menopause keep estrogen from being more widely prescribed. Another medication, Evista (*raloxifene*), acts like estrogen in the bones and uterus, while blocking estrogen's effect in breast tissue. For post-menopausal women who have had a hysterectomy, Evista can be used to maintain normal bone density and as a preventative measure for breast cancer. It has other side effects, however, including an increased risk of forming blood clots.

The adult bone of men similarly is developed and maintained under the influence of the male hormone, testosterone. Although the decline in testosterone production in older men is not as abrupt as menopause in females, it is steady. By the time men reach their early 80s, most are showing both a measurable decline in testosterone and a corresponding decline in bone density. Many men in their 80s and older have osteoporosis as a result. Testosterone can be used to improve osteoporosis in men but more often the other, non-sex hormone treatments are recommended.

Finally, there is a mineral, *strontium*, that has been shown in many studies to increase bone density and reduce fracture risk. Strontium is naturally available in ground surface water. Prior to the 20th century, all human bones included a significant level of strontium in addition to calcium. Even for those who lived into their 70s and beyond, there were very few cases of osteoporosis. Unfortunately, virtually all the processes we now use to purify water for drinking also remove strontium. In Europe, one of the drug companies developed a form of strontium called *strontium renalate* which has been shown to reduce and reverse the loss of bone density and strength seen in osteoporosis. The results have been significant enough that the other medications listed above are used much less frequently in Europe than in the United States. Recently, however, the safety of strontium renalate has been called into question because of an increase in vascular disease in those for whom it has been prescribed. Evidence seems to support the idea that renalic acid, which is manmade, is the likely culprit. Strontium renalate has never been approved for prescription in the United States.

There is a common salt of strontium that is available over the counter in the United States (and elsewhere as well). This is *strontium citrate*. Recent studies of strontium citrate at several American medical schools have demonstrated both its effectiveness and safety in dealing with osteoporosis. The effective daily dose of strontium citrate is 680 mg of elemental calcium (1944 mg of strontium citrate). It needs to be taken on an empty stomach and at least a couple of hours apart from taking calcium or magnesium.

JOINTS

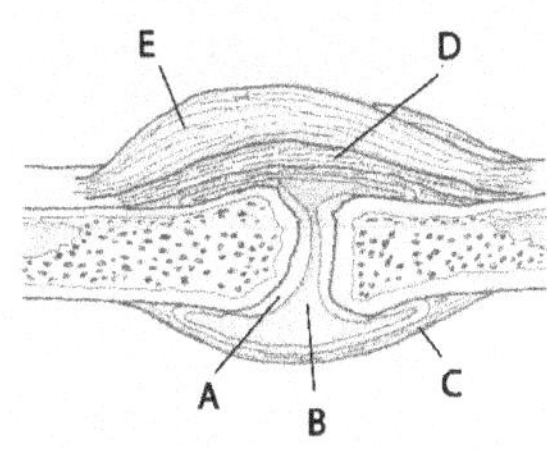

Fig. 2-3:
Joint internal structure
A: joint surface cartilage;
B: joint space;
C: fluid producing
  membrane (Synovial
  membrane);
D: joint capsule;
E: external ligament.

Joints allow a connection between two bones so that they can move relative to each other. A healthy joint consists of two surfaces between two bones. These surfaces most frequently are on rounded heads and are cupped receiving surfaces generally located at or near the end of the bones. Each surface of the two bones where they meet is covered by cartilage, a form of connective tissue that is both smooth and somewhat flexible. By covering the surface of the boney joint where the bones could potentially come into contact with each other during movement (Fig. 2-3), cartilage provides a smooth, slick surface. Between the two cartilage-covered surfaces is joint fluid made up of water, electrolytes (minerals) and proteins. Joint fluid is thicker than blood and enhances the slick interface between the two cartilage surfaces. Recall that the joint capsule is a bag of tough connective tissue enclosing the joint. The joint capsule includes specialized tissue on its inner surface that generates and absorbs the joint fluid as needed. The joint capsule also keeps that joint fluid from escaping the joint.

MUSCLES

Muscle cells generate most, if not all, of the movement in our bodies (Fig. 2-4a). Each muscle cell has many parallel bands of *actin* and *myosin* that act as ratchet motors energized by the molecule *adenosine triphosphate* (ATP). As the *actin-myosin* contracts, so does the corresponding muscle cell, and when it relaxes the muscle cell does, too. Typically, muscle cells

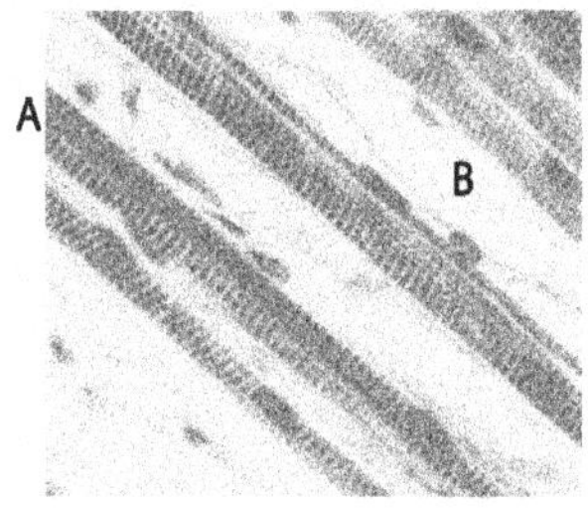

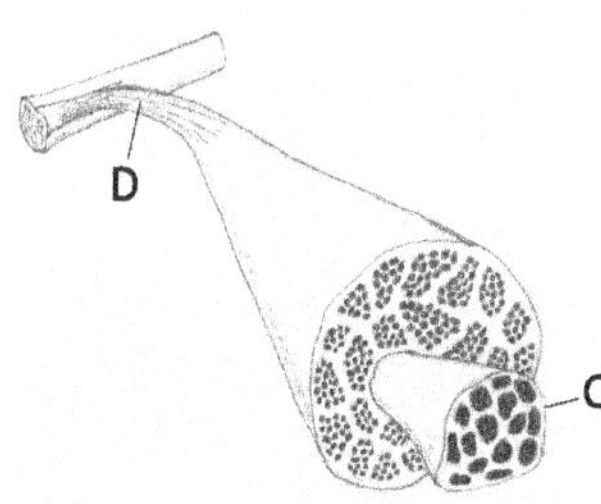

Fig. 2-4:
A: Skeletal muscle cell;
B: Fascia surrounding
  muscle cells;
C: muscle fascicles;
D: tendon attaching
  muscle to bone.

are attached to each other and to local connective tissue (Fig. 2-4b). The muscle cells are activated and begin to contract because an electric or chemical signal opens microscopic pores in the cell surface and sodium, potassium and calcium ions cross the membrane. If there is too much calcium or potassium outside the cell, the contractions are prolonged and uncontrolled. Too little and the muscle cells won't contract at all. When muscle cells contract, the distance between their ends shortens but they become thicker. When most of the muscle cells in a particular muscle shorten, the whole muscle bulges in the middle.

Even though muscle cells connect to each other, in order to have something to pull on they attach to a scaffold of connective tissue (Fig. 2-4c). Without that matrix, individual muscle cells and even groups of muscle cells could not produce any meaningful movement in our bodies. With the connective tissue, the contraction of muscle cells produces the possibility of movement.

The typical muscle cell communicates with its immediate neighbors so that if one begins to contract, its neighbor will, too. If one begins to relax, its neighbors follow suit. Thus, in any group of muscle cells we see waves of contraction followed by waves of relaxation.

Muscle cells come in three basic types:

The skeletal muscle cells are bound together in elongated groups called *fascicles* (Fig. 2-4c). Each fascicle is surrounded by connective tissue. The connective tissue then binds many fascicles together to form a muscle. Surrounding the muscle is denser connective tissue. The connective tissue comes together in a tough, fibrous band called a tendon (Fig 2-4d). These tendons at either end of the muscle then attach to different bones. When the muscle contracts, it pulls the two bones closer together (as can be seen in Fig. 2-5b). Skeletal muscles are the source of body movement and the focus of this book. Skeletal muscle cells typically require stimulation from the central nervous system (brain and spinal cord) to cause their activation.

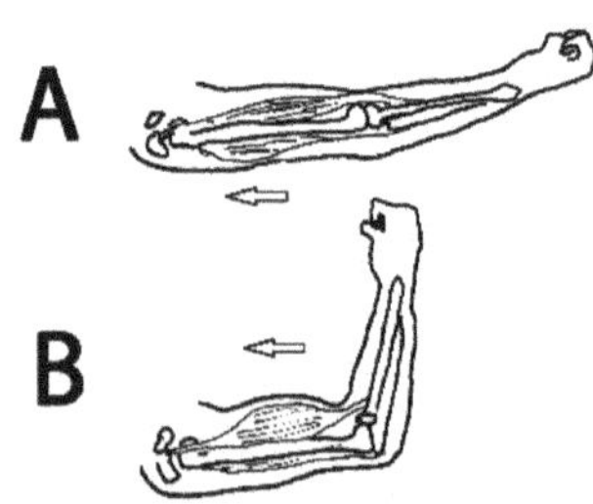

Fig. 2-5: Muscle contraction draws two bones into
A: an extended relationship;
B: a flexed relationship.

Smooth muscle cells are found in the internal organs, arteries and glands and produce the internal movements of the organs, glands and tension/relaxation in the arteries. They are not banded together in thick groups, but typically form thin sheets. Smooth muscle cells may operate based on internally generated waves of activation but are generally somewhat controlled by groups of autonomic nervous system cells (*ganglia*). Smooth muscle cells and the autonomic ganglia typically operate independently from the central nervous system although their activity can be influenced by the brain and spinal cord.

Heart muscle cells: Intermediate between these two types are the heart muscle cells. Heart muscle is quite thick and strong, but contracts based on its own internal rhythm, much like smooth muscle cells. Interestingly anatomists have discovered that the heart is a single long thick sheet of muscle that coils and wraps on itself to create and enclose the chambers for the blood that needs to be pumped. (See Gerald Buckhorn, "Unwrapping the Heart, Part 1" on vimeo.com)

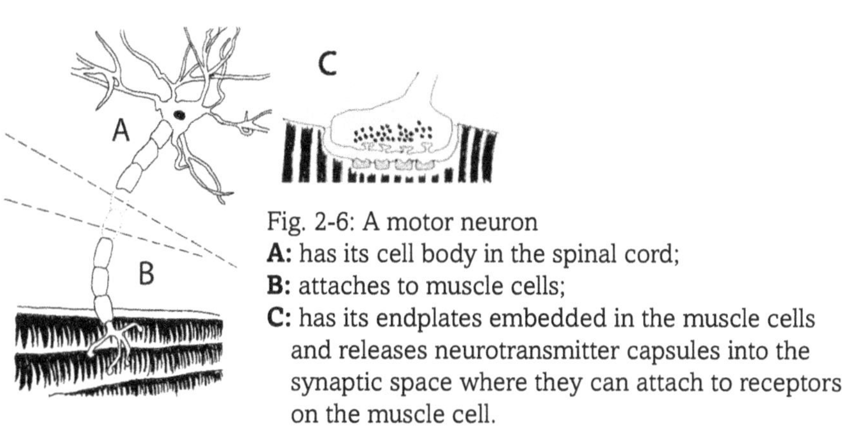

Fig. 2-6: A motor neuron
A: has its cell body in the spinal cord;
B: attaches to muscle cells;
C: has its endplates embedded in the muscle cells and releases neurotransmitter capsules into the synaptic space where they can attach to receptors on the muscle cell.

MOTOR NERVES

The signal to make a skeletal muscle contract comes from the large and fast conducting motor neurons. Motor in this case refers to the processes that lead to movement. A motor neuron has its cell body in the brainstem or spinal cord (central nervous system) (Fig.2-6a), but sends a long fiber, an *axon,* out to the muscle (Fig. 2-6b). A number of these axons are bundled together into a nerve that comes from a specific place in the brainstem or spinal cord. When the nerve penetrates the outer layer of the muscle connective tissue, it divides into many fine finger–like projections that connect to muscle cell bundles. The actual terminations have miscroscopic gaps between the nerve endings and the muscle. (Fig. 2-6c). When a nerve signal (electrical impulse) comes down from the central nervous system, the nerve ending releases a tiny amount of a chemical called *acetylcholine.* This chemical binds to receptors on the muscle side of the gap. When *acetylcholine* binds to the muscle receptors a complex bioelectric cascade is set in motion that causes the muscle cells to contract. If the motor nerve is cut to a particular muscle the immediate result is that the muscle is unable to move. If the motor nerve does not regrow, the muscle cells will die and the muscle will waste away.

The motor neuron is in turn driven by a complex set of neurons coming from the brain cortex, the midbrain, the cerebellum, the brainstem and other parts of the spinal cord. These command centers trigger and coordinate the movement of multiple muscles in order to generate the complex ballet of movement that allows us to do such complex things as sit, walk, exercise and even write this book.

BOTOX

There is a toxin or poison from a bacterium called Clostridium botulinum that is among the most powerful available. Botulinum toxin produces a long-term blockade of acetylcholine release, preventing muscle contraction. If it gets into our general circulation, it will cause rapid death by paralysis. A common name for the disease caused by this bacterium and its toxin is "lock jaw" or tetanus. However medical science has tamed this once common disease by immunization (tetanus vaccine or Td vaccine). Medical science has even bent the toxin into something useful in neurological and muscular disease, and even cosmetic treatment in the form of Botox.

SENSORY NERVES AND THE SOMA

In order to properly manage the muscles, the central nervous system also receives sensory information from the muscles, tendons, ligaments, joints and bones. These sensory nerves have endings embedded in the muscles, tendons, ligaments, joint capsules as well as in the connective tissue throughout the body. In the muscles, tendons, ligaments and joint capsules there are sensory endings that respond to the velocity, acceleration and force of muscle contraction, the stress(es) placed on the connective tissue and to potentially destructive forces occurring in the tissue.

Most of these sensors have to do with coordinating the action of muscles. These proprioceptors involve fast conducting neurons that provide feedback at multiple levels in the central nervous system. Another class of sensory neurons, the pain receptors respond to potential damaging events and will be discussed in greater detail in coming chapters. The pain receptor sensory endings are found only in connective tissue and never within the muscle cell bundles.

THE MOVEMENT UNIT

Let's look at a joint and its muscles. Our model joint is a simple ball and socket. In fact, no such simple joints exist in our body. However, to understand the basic principles of movement we will start with this simple model. Two long bones are joined by a ball and socket. The possible range of motion would be determined by how shallow or deep the socket is. For our purposes, we will assume that the motion is only in two dimensions. Because of the position of the cup, the bone with the ball can move from a position with shafts parallel (Fig. 2-5a) to a position with the shafts a bit more than 90 degrees to each other (Fig. 2-5b). On the upper side we find a muscle that has its tendons attached to the upper side of both long bones. When the upper muscle contracts, it brings the bones into the 90-degree position (Fig. 2-5b). If it relaxes, the bones can line up with each other. The joint will be straight. In order to bring the bones back into the lined-up position we place another muscle on the underside of the bones. When the top muscle contracts, the lower muscle is stretched. When the lower muscle contracts, the upper muscle is stretched. If we send the central nervous system a signal for each muscle to relax when its opponent contracts, we have a simple movement.

We see something very like this simple arrangement of opposing muscles in our fingers, elbows and knees although the joints are more complex by having two balls and sockets at the ends of the bone. This is how motion is kept largely in one plane. Across these long bone joints the muscles that bring the joint straight to 180 degrees are termed extensors and those that bring the joint to 90 degrees are termed flexors. A great way to see this simple muscle unit at work is the deep tendon reflex doctors try to elicit when they tap your knee with a reflex hammer. In the knee, the extensor tendon is relaxed when the joint is flexed. By tapping on the extensor tendon (for the quadriceps muscle) the sensory information is sent to the spinal cord that stimulates the quadriceps along the front of the thigh to contract. At the same time the flexors (hamstrings on the back of the thigh) relax. This causes the knee to straighten out or extend. Since the sensory feedback is not persistent the next stage is that the hamstrings contact and the quadriceps relaxes, bringing the knee back into flexion.

In most of the joints of the body a similar arrangement exists with muscles that are generally active when their opposing muscle is relaxed. Some joints have multi-dimensional motions like the hip and shoulder and will therefore have more than two opposing muscle pairs around the joint. Other joints may have muscles that cross at an angle, causing the joint to twist.

THE DYNAMIC BODY

Our bodies have many of these opposing pairs of muscles around many joints. In order to function we must be able to do more than merely bend or straighten a particular joint. We must be able to move many joints at once in a coordinated fashion. Taking a simple step requires activation and then inactivation of most of the joints of the body, some simultaneously and some in sequence. Even more remarkable, we do this without giving it a moment's thought. The same part of the brain that allows us to learn the movements for a dance routine or a new sport are involved in developing, learning, maintaining and coordinating all these complex movements we use without even thinking. This is the role of our cerebellum, which is found at the base of the brain.

The coordinated patterns required for walking or simply reaching for and picking something up are very complex. We may decide to get up from the chair where we are reading this and walk into the kitchen to get a glass of water but the movements themselves are complex beyond comprehension. Even more remarkable, unlike most animals, we stand and walk on only two feet. Incredible!

Even the process of simply standing still requires ongoing activation and inactivation of many muscles. The act of breathing expands and contracts our chest and changes our center of gravity. Try standing on your toes with your eyes closed. You will quickly become aware of how you are shifting your weight as you breathe.

The nervous system acts as the controller and coordinator of these muscles. We need functional sensory inputs to tell the nervous system how well things are moving, where the muscles and joints are in relation to their potential range of motion, what kind of surface is under our feet, whether we are upright or tilted, and where other things are in space. When any of these elements is less than optimal or fails altogether our ability to move becomes compromised. An ankle sprain causes us to decrease the amount of weight we put on the injured ankle. The way we walk and stand is altered. We limp, which is significantly less efficient, and we find ourselves running out of steam more easily. We may find that we develop pain elsewhere too, such as in the shoulder or neck. If we have the skill and knowledge of where and how to look, we will note other more subtle signs of restriction in the pelvis, spine, chest, shoulders and neck. Our normal easy dynamic motion has been altered. In fact, it has been degraded. We can still function, although in a compromised fashion. Where before we might have been able to run, now we only limp along. And yet, our system is so robust and adaptive that we can still walk.

Consider the case of one of my patients. He was a vigorous, 39-year-old male who was quite active in sports including running year around and playing baseball during the summer. He had never had any musculoskeletal injuries or problems until three months before he came to see me. He had not fallen, but somehow had developed severe low back pain the day after playing in a 10-inning baseball game. He tried ibuprofen and ice and then heat. When his pain did not resolve after a couple of days he went to a walk-in clinic near where he lived. X-rays taken there did not show anything abnormal, so they gave him prescriptions for hydrocodone and a muscle relaxer and sent him to an orthopedic spine surgeon. The surgeon ordered an MRI and when the results came back with no pathology my patient was sent to physical therapy. Although the surgeon was willing to leave him on the muscle relaxer, he told him no further narcotics would be prescribed because the problem was not structural. Instead, he gave him a prescription for 800 mg of ibuprofen three times a day. He was instructed to lay off running and baseball until the physical therapist cleared him for normal activity.

Unfortunately, physical therapy did little to change this patient's pain. He began to gain weight because of the enforced inactivity. Even worse, he began to develop pain in his right groin which interfered with his sexual activity. He tried to start walking daily but couldn't walk more than 10-15 minutes. After a failed trial of acupuncture, he finally came to see me on the advice of a friend.

When I first saw this patient, he was limping and his right shoulder was visibly lower than the left. His right hip was shifted to the right and he had developed a sideways curve to his lower back. He told me he had never had a curvature in his low back, or any of his spine, for that matter. As I examined him on the table, I found his right ribs were bent down toward the table when he was seated. When he laid on his back on the table it quickly became apparent that his right hip was higher than his left. In fact, his right leg appeared to be an inch and a half shorter than his left. He was told what my findings were and, with his consent, I began to treat him starting with the rib strains and then for the upwardly shifted right half of his pelvis. The left half of his pelvis was also shifted downward. After treatment, his rib strains resolved and there was no leg length difference even when he stood. His pain was gone and after a couple of days to allow his system to settle he was able to return to baseball. He began walking and then after a week or two, running. We never did identify exactly what had happened to cause him such grief.

If one thinks about it, my patient had been walking as if he had a 1 ½ inch block (like a piece of wood) under one foot. His walking was not comfortable, but he was able to stand and walk. He did not fall over, but it was clear that his somatic compensation left him neither pain-free nor as capable of activity as it had been before his problem developed.

BALANCE AND COORDINATED FUNCTION

Perhaps we might consider what happens with balance. As young people, we typically do not give much thought to the problems of simply standing or walking without falling. But as we age, simply staying on our feet can become a problem. I remember a description of the problem of balance as being like a four-legged stool. One leg is our vision. One leg is the vestibular body in our inner ear. And two legs are the skin and *proprioceptor* sensations from our feet and legs. The brain puts information from all four of these sensory systems together and issues instructions to the muscles that allow us to stand and walk. If vision fails, we still have three legs to stand on. If the vestibular apparatus gives poorly coordinated information, we may be dizzy. We will be able to stand and walk, but our balance may be precarious. If we lose sensory information from both our feet as commonly occurs in neuropathy, we can't feel the ground we are walking on. If we lose any two of these systems, we are under constant threat of falling. And if we lose all three, as may occur at an advanced age, we literally do not have a leg to stand on.

Consider how much of a problem a new stroke victim has trying to reestablish balanced patterns of movement. In most cases, this redevelopment of complex movement seems to be harder than it was when he first learned them as an infant. Part of the brain is missing and the brain and body have to learn new ways of achieving normal function.

CONNECTIVE TISSUE AND "MEMORY"

We normally associate learning and memory with our nervous system. However, connective tissue has its own form of memory that plays a significant role in the maintenance of and recovery from pain. This is termed elastic memory.

Suppose you have a rubber tire on a car that is sitting, unmoving, out in the hot summer sun for several days. If you get in the car and start to slowly drive off, you may notice a thumping sound that comes from the tires. This occurs because the tires have developed a flat spot where they were sitting on the pavement. After driving a short while, the thumping will disappear because the flat spots have been rounded out by the heat created by friction and movement. If you stop the car, get out and jack up one of the corners of the car so a tire is suspended in the air, the tire will be perfectly round. Now, if you hit the tire with a hammer the flat spot will reappear. This is what is termed elastic memory. It is a property of rubber and other flexible materials. Energy applied while the flexible material is in a deformed state results in a memory of the deformed state. Another application of energy, such as stretching the material, may restore it to apparent normalcy. However, the memory is still there and the deformity can be easily retriggered.

Both fascia and bone show elastic memory. Recall that fascia is the soft "skeleton" for all our organs. It wraps around and provides a mesh structure within our muscles so the actual muscle cells can have something to pull on when they contract. It ties the ends of muscles to bones. It provides the capsules around the joints between bones. It is the ligaments between bones that stabilize our joints. Bone is the hard skeleton of the body. Because bone is based in connective tissue, even with its hard calcium inclusion, bone demonstrates elastic memory.

When we experience an event that involves force enough to deform our tissues, it may also induce an elastic memory in those tissues that reinforces that deformity. For instance, one of the common complaints I encounter in my medical practice is a pain involving the upper back under the shoulder blade. One such patient had been driving a car. His car was hit on the driver's side and he fell to his right. He came to see me six weeks later after an Emergency Room visit, X-rays, a visit to his primary physician and five weeks of physical therapy. He had unexplained pain under his right shoulder blade that was causing him problems with breathing and in using his arm.

There was no visible evidence of trauma to his right shoulder and his lungs sounded normal. He did have an upward shear of his right hip, like the last case discussed. Causing him the most pain were ribs 3, 4, and 5 on his right side which had been strained. Recall that bones are flexible. The ribs themselves are quite flexible allowing us to expand and contract our chest during breathing. The type of strain in this patient's three right ribs involved a compression deformity of the ribs from the side. The front ends were pushed forward, and back angles pushed backward. This mild deformity was easily palpated but could not be seen on X-rays. Since these ribs run under the shoulder blade and most of the muscle of the shoulder attaches to them, the deformity affected the use of his shoulder and arm. The patient felt like there was a rock under his shoulder blade.

Manual therapy in the form of osteopathic manipulative therapy was sufficient to restore the ribs to a more normal presentation and shape. The muscles and tendons around the ribs could then be restored to normal function. The patient walked out of the office feeling pain-free for the first time since his accident.

Two weeks later he returned for his follow-up. Although he had some discomfort in his right hip and neck, his chest and shoulder remained pain free and there was no sign of his rib strain. At a planned follow-up three weeks later, however, he again complained about his right chest and shoulder pain. On questioning, he had an allergy attack four days prior to this visit and had spent a couple of days coughing and sneezing. The pain in his ribs had returned as he was coughing. Structurally the same three ribs, 3, 4, and 5 showed the same strain pattern they had five weeks ago when he was first seen. Although he had not suffered any further falls or injuries, the force of his cough had been enough to trigger the elastic memory of his ribs and the joints, ligaments, muscles, and tendons around these ribs. Manual treatment was successful in reducing his pain. He has not had problems with those ribs since.

One of the working models for many of those who come to see someone like me for persistent musculoskeletal pain is that we must work to reduce memory of the painful event. Obviously, we must consider mental memories and their consequences and any pain-related reflexes, both of which involve the nervous system. We must also consider the fascial memory when we are trying to get rid of pain. In each form of memory, we are trying to help the body and brain find "normal" again and put the memories of trauma away. If the original trauma was great or the time in which it remained untreated was long, it will take time, patience and frequent reintroduction of normal physical and mental balance to reduce the trauma memories.

CHAPTER 3
Somatic Injury, Inflammation and Healing

A typical somatic injury starts with force introduced into an out-of-balance body. This could be something as obvious as a fall or a motor vehicle accident. It could be something less obvious like bending the wrong way, or stepping down a step unexpectedly, or even tripping or stumbling without falling.

Sometimes the injury is not so much due to the force, but instead is due to prolonged positioning in an out-of-balance state. This can include a wide variety of things including falling asleep slumped to one side in a chair, sitting and watching a TV that is not right in front of you or working for a prolonged period under a sink which could only be reached by contorting the body.

Such events occur frequently in our daily living and for the most part we do not notice them nor do we seem to suffer from any prolonged ill-effects. This is because, in most cases, the body can spontaneously correct for any changes that these events have caused either immediately or overnight. Being young and staying physically active so that the body is strong and flexible seems to help the spontaneous recovery from injuries. When events trigger a longer-lasting imbalance in the body it will require effort and sometimes physical intervention to overcome.

To understand what an injury does and why it may require intervention, we need to look at the underlying mechanisms involved in both the injury and the healing.

THE PAIN RECEPTOR

Pain receptors start in the tissues as specialized sensors called free nerve endings. These nerve endings are branched out in the tissue, like a root system of a tree. Pain receptors are found in most tissues of the body, particularly the fascia. Pain receptors respond to potentially injurious happenings. In biology and medicine, these sensory neurons are termed *nociceptors*. However, we will use the terms pain receptors or pain sensory neurons. The tissue event that triggers the pain sensory neurons into action can involve twisting, cutting, tearing, breaking, burning, freezing, compression, distension, loss of blood supply, lack of enough oxygen, lack of nutrients, or abnormal chemistry. When the free nerve endings of these pain receptors are stimulated by damage or potential damage, they send signals to the spinal cord and brain and into the many other "roots" of the same nerve spread throughout the tissue.

When these pain signals enter the central nervous system, they can trigger multiple responses. They can stimulate the motor neurons that will cause muscle activation. They can stimulate the sympathetic neurons that will cause arousal and the fight, flight, or fright response. Or they can send signals up the long pathways to the brain where they stimulate emotional responses. If these signals reach the cortex of the brain, we become aware of the pain.

INJURY REFLEXES

Many body responses to pain are entirely involuntary. Pain-related muscle reflexes can occur even when there is no conscious awareness and maybe even when we are attempting to block them. The classic version of this occurs when an arm or a leg is given a strong and sudden painful input like burning heat or cold, an electrical shock, or a piercing of the skin by a thorn, needle or broken piece of glass. The limb is withdrawn involuntarily, often with a jerk.

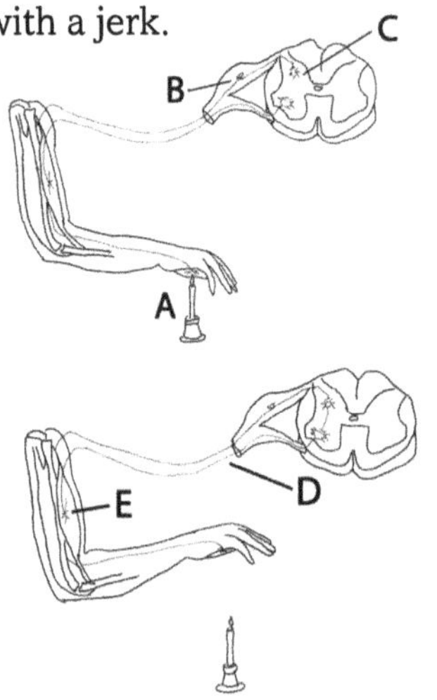

Fig. 3-1: Pain withdrawal reflex.
A: a painful stimulus (flame applied to the palm of the hand) triggers
B: pain signal in a pain sensory neuron;
C: the pain sensory neuron stimulates
D: a short interneuron in the spinal cord;
E: the spinal interneuron triggers a motor neuron in the spinal cord to send a signal to a flexor muscle;
F: the flexor muscle contracts moving the limb away from the painful stimulus.

The mechanism for these pain withdrawal reflexes is quite simple (Fig.3-1). When the pain nerves enter the spinal cord or brainstem they terminate (*synapse*) on the next level of neurons. Some of the receiving neurons connect to motor neurons in the spinal cord and brainstem. Recall that these motor neurons have *axons* (fibers) that leave the spinal cord or brainstem and go to the muscles. Remember when motor neurons activate, they cause the muscles to contract. This pathway from the *pain receptor* to processing neuron and then to the motor neuron is the basis of the reflex response to pain, like jerking away from a pin prick or a flame. This is the withdrawal reflex.

Coupled with these immediate withdrawal reflexes are another set that minimizes further pain by limiting use of the affected body part. The classic demonstration of this reflex is seen in a dog with a bur in its paw. The affected leg is lifted at its attachment to the body and the dog walks on the other three legs. This is not a conscious decision on the dog's part. Instead, it is a complex reflex organized in the spinal cord. We show similar use-limiting reflexes. If we burn our fingers, we tend not to use them until the burn is healed. We cannot, however, totally disable a leg with an injury and still walk. Instead, there is a reflex shortening of the injured leg at the hip that can almost always be demonstrated when the person is asked to lie on their back. We can still walk, but our gait is no longer entirely normal or balanced.

PAIN AND INFLAMMATION

Pain is the result of injury or potential injury. It and the associated inflammation are a part of the body's protective response. When there is tissue damage, we typically see a cascade of reactions that start with the pain fibers being triggered. This tissue cascade is the result of pain fibers releasing a stew of chemicals into the injured tissue at the same time they are sending pain signals toward the central nervous system. These local chemicals cause the tissue to swell and redden, a reaction we term inflammation. We tend to think of pain and inflammation as something to be avoided. In fact, we spend a lot of time and money in our medical system trying to prevent and reverse both pain and inflammation because they are portrayed as being so undesirable. However, pain and inflammation also play critical roles in healing from injury.

PAIN AND HEALING

When the pain receptors to a specific tissue are not there, the healing response is seriously delayed or blocked. Experimental studies with animal models showed this long ago. If the pain nerves to an animal's foot were destroyed and the foot is then injured by simply making a small cut in the skin, it would take much longer for the wound to heal even if it was kept in a sterile condition. In some cases, it would not heal at all. Instead, it would develop a skin ulcer. If it was not kept completely sterile it would quickly become infected.

We see the same thing in human beings who have lost the pain receptors in a particular tissue. For instance, diabetics commonly develop a problem termed peripheral neuropathy after years of dealing with the disease. The nerves in the feet and eventually in the lower legs and hands die back. This includes not only the sensory nerves for touch but also those for pain. The nerve die-back can go so far that there is almost no sensation in the feet, whether to touch, heat, cold, or pin prick. If there is any injury to that person's foot, it will be very slow to heal and it may not heal at all. Although some of the failure to heal is clearly due to decreased circulation, the lack of pain nerves to initiate the healing response also plays a significant role.

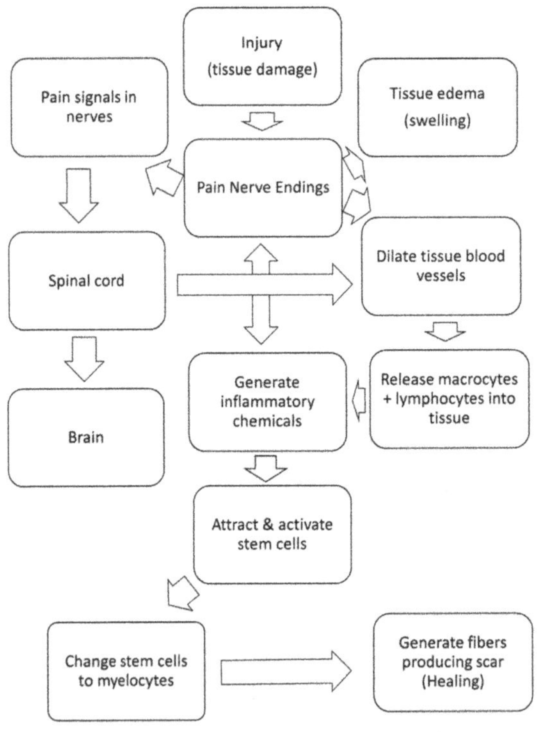

Fig. 3-2: Inflammation and healing.

INFLAMMATION AND HEALING

When there is tissue damage, we should see a cascade of body reactions that we call inflammation. Inflammation starts with the pain caused by nerve endings releasing chemicals into the very tissues that have been injured (Fig. 3-2).

These chemicals cause the tissue to swell and redden, one of the first signs of inflammation. There is an increase in local tissue fluid, called edema. If the tissue is near the surface of the skin there may be a reddening of the skin, called *erythema*. This reddening is due to dilation of the small blood vessels within and overlying the tissue. The local tissue temperature also increases.

Dilation of the capillaries and other small blood vessels leads to increased flow of fluid across the blood vessel walls into the surrounding tissue. Dilation of the blood vessels also allows blood-borne white blood cells to move into the tissue. The white blood cells include macrophages and lymphocytes which help clear the area of damaged and dead cells and fibers. They also generate chemicals that further dilate blood vessels in the area to carry nutrients into the tissue and debris away. Some of these chemicals also stimulate the pain receptors. The chemicals attract stem cells into the tissues that will change physically, allowing the tissue to be rebuilt. Thus, the tissue can go through the process we call healing.

It is likely that much of the failure to heal when pain receptors are absent is due to the failure to initiate the inflammatory response. Likewise, there is evidence that when the inflammatory processes are too vigorously blocked, healing may be slowed or may even fail.

Because prolonged inflammation and pain have their own negative effects on us physically and psychologically, as stated before we tend to focus on the elimination of both. Sometimes we do so immediately at the onset of pain, even though we may be interfering with healing. Of course, prolonged and uncontrolled inflammation can have significant negative effects on health and healing as seen in many autoimmune diseases. However, blocking pain and inflammation in acute injury should be done carefully and perhaps even avoided.

Normally healing occurs in stages. Whether the tissue is the skin, the underlying connective tissue or bone, the first stage is inflammation that peaks at about two days. It is during this stage that the blood volume to the tissue increases and the macrophages and lymphocytes from the blood are delivered to the injured tissue. Next stem cells from the blood and the tissue evolve into specialized cells called myofibroblasts. These cells produce connective fibers in a random matrix that we call scar tissue when it matures. For some tissues this can develop in as little as three weeks. If the injury involves a sprain of the tendons or ligaments, it will take about four weeks for the injury to heal. If it is a broken bone, healing will generally take between four and six weeks because the process also involves setting calcium into the connective tissue matrix (scar).

These immediate responses to tissue damage are the start of the healing response. If the tissue is restored to a relatively normal position the healing will allow near-normal function. If healing occurs with the tissue in an abnormal position, that position and limited range of motion will put the tissue under persistent stress. Any additional stress to this tissue results in persistent inflammation as tissue fibers are overstressed and damaged requiring the healing to begin again. The inflammation in on-going stressed tissue can often be felt as tissue bogginess, abnormal firmness, stiffness or laxity, and difference in color and temperature (warmer or sometimes even cooler).

SCAR TISSUE FROM DISUSE

Total disuse of a piece of fascia also leads to what amounts to replacement of normally organized tissue with something that resembles scar tissue. Recall that fascia is always regenerating. Most of the time the regeneration is along the lines of stress (Fig. 3-3a). When fascia is immobilized, the normal stresses are removed. As a result, the ongoing regeneration begins to generate fibers in a random meshwork resembling scar tissue (Fig. 3-3b).

A 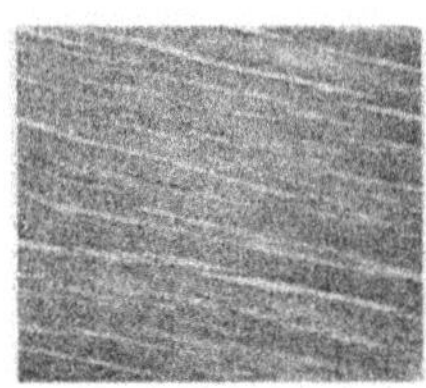 B 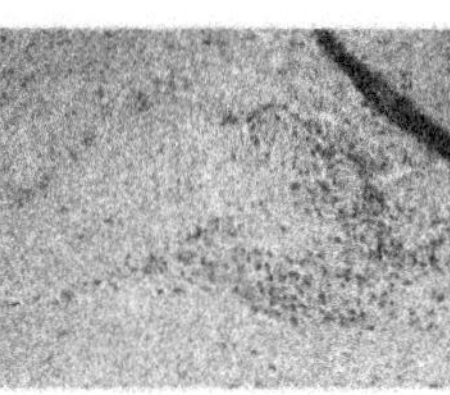

Fig 3-3:
A: normal connective tissue organized along lines of stress;
B: scar tissue disorganized and random.

This random meshwork cannot take the normal load. Worse yet, the tissue may shorten and become less dense. A tissue that might have been an inch long might now be only 2/3 of an inch long. The tissue may also become thicker because the random assortment of fibers is no longer organized in a tight bundle. The result is that the tissue is no longer flexible and strong. Under a load that it might have handled easily when healthy, the tissue now may be more easily torn. At the same time, attempting to move the immobilized tissue will trigger tearing and activation of pain receptors, causing us to limit movement.

MOTION RESTRICTION

Tissues that heal in an abnormal position always show a decreased range of motion. The classical extremes of such a limitation are the frozen shoulder or frozen finger joint. More frequently there is a decrease in the available motion of a tissue without total restriction. If a wrist is injured and its bones, muscles and connective tissues heal before those tissues are restored to their normal positions, we may see a decrease of available motion from about 125 degrees combined flexion and extension to about 70 degrees combined flexion and extension. Attempts to exceed this restricted range are accompanied by pain. We don't like pain so we don't push beyond this new normal.

REORGANIZATION OF SCAR TISSUE WITH USE

One of the remarkable properties of our healing response is that the development of scar tissue is not the end of the process. The body has the capacity to remodel scar tissue over time. To understand this process, we need to go back to the nature of a scar. In scar tissue, the myofibroblasts have produced their fibers in random orientations. They will not be oriented in a linear fashion even when the original tissue was linear, such as in a tendon or ligament. Production of enough of these randomly oriented fibers and the hole in the tissue is filled up. Healing is complete.

However, the scar tissue will be chronically or even periodically pulled in a particular direction like the original tissue. Those fibers laid out in a direction other than that of the pulling will tend to be broken. Every time some of these off-axis fibers are torn or broken, the inflammatory and healing process begins again. Myofibroblasts start generating new fibers. Remembering that all fascia tends to be reorganized along the lines of stress, we can see that over time the scar tissue becomes organized along the line of pull as the off-axis fibers are repeatedly broken and more on-axis fibers are laid down. Eventually most of the fibers in what used to be a scar are laid down along the lines of stress and what was scar tissue now looks and functions very much like the original connective tissue. A similar process occurs in bone following a fracture.

STRUCTURAL IMBALANCE AND COMPENSATION

When there is an injury, the effects are not limited to the local tissue that is obviously damaged. Let's start with a simple example. You twist and sprain your ankle. We are going to assume you do not fall and nothing is broken. There is immediate tissue swelling and inflammation accompanied by pain in the ankle. You may be able to walk on the foot but you will consciously and unconsciously walk in a way to minimize further damage and pain. In other words, you limp. That means when you walk and stand, the other leg will carry most of your weight. As discussed above, your foot will not be moved as much and the period it actually spends on the ground will be less than normal. You will probably show a shortening of the injured leg at the hip as we discussed before. Your pelvis and sacrum will no longer be level. This tends to bend the spine to one side. To keep from falling over, the spine above will bend in the opposite direction. Such sideways curves are termed scoliosis and may be subtle or quite pronounced. The shoulders become unleveled and the neck may even develop a tilt. All of these changes occurred because you sprained your ankle.

These changes in widespread parts of the body because of localized injury are called compensation. These compensatory responses are rarely voluntary or planned. For the most part they are driven by unconscious management of our muscles, although we may be aware of their consequences. These processes are like those that occur when you try to stand on one foot. You are not aware of all the neural and muscle interactions that take place when you try to stand on one foot, but you are aware that it takes effort, and you are particularly aware when you lose your balance.

The cascade of compensatory changes that occur from local injury is not fixed. Rather it is a dynamic and ongoing process that occurs as you try to use a system that is no longer completely balanced. Muscles that normally would go quiet during part of our activity now are more chronically active. Other muscles may fail to act when they should. A task that is normally effortless suddenly requires effort. Efforts that were painless may cause pain, and not always at the site of the injury. We may continue to function, but we are no longer working at our best.

SLEEP AND HEALING

Sleep is necessary for a variety of reasons that are best seen when it is disturbed. That sleep is necessary for our mental well-being is best demonstrated when people are intentionally deprived of all sleep. After three or more days of sleep deprivation the person may exhibit psychotic-like states with hallucinations and very disturbed mental and emotional states. While sleep disturbance that allows some daily sleep does not produce such dramatic effects, most people show increasing irritability, decreasing mental acuity and reaction times, a tendency to fall asleep at inappropriate times, and delayed or poor physical healing. The effect of poor sleep on healing is strong because sleep is the time when most of the healing from injury occurs.

Pain can be a major factor in producing sleep disturbance. Pain is essentially arousing. If it occurs when we are trying to sleep it can interfere with developing the relaxing body and brain rhythms of sleep. Pain can delay the onset of sleep because most of us have to be reasonably comfortable to get to sleep in the first place. If the pain is intense enough it becomes a focus for attention and may send us into the spiral of worrying about whether we will get to sleep at all. These worries delay sleep, too. Even when we get to sleep, pain can break the cycle early. Sometimes this early awakening will be later in the sleep cycle but it can occur after only an hour or two. Again, once awakened to pain, returning to sleep can be difficult. We fight the pain and its arousal and worry about getting back to sleep. We worry whether we will be able to get enough sleep before we need to get up.

The worst issue with poor sleep quality is that it can also amplify or even cause pain. One of the best examples is the problem called fibromyalgia. In this case, poor quality sleep and lack of sleep triggers pain in muscles all over our body. Restoring good quality and appropriate amounts of sleep will often cause the muscle pains to disappear.

CHAPTER 4
Fascia

We all remember the advice from our coaches in high school, college or our drill sergeant in the military: "No pain, no gain." It is true in most cases that exercise in itself often produces pain at least for short periods. This pain can come from tendons and joint capsules that are tighter than the particular activity requires. It can also be from muscles that are being worked harder than they have been in the past. Neither form of pain is long-term, nor is it severe enough to override the drive to improve the way we feel.

A similar piece of advice from our coaches has always been "use it or lose it." Muscles, tendons, ligaments and joint capsules respond to use and disuse. We all know that the way to make a muscle stronger and, in some cases, larger, is to make it work repeatedly against a load. Under repetitive loads the muscle fibers actually divide to produce more muscle cells. Use also strengthens the action of each muscle cell over time.

We also know what happens to muscles when they aren't used. Quite simply, they become weaker. If we have worked hard to build muscle strength, size, and stamina but then through circumstance or laziness stop working out, the muscles shrink and weaken. When we are young this process is relatively slow. Unfortunately, as we age the losses are more rapid with inactivity and regaining strength takes longer. Think about how small an arm is after six weeks of immobilization in a cast for a broken wrist. The bellies of the muscles are small, tight and ropey. The joints that were immobilized in the cast are stiff and hard to move. The tendons are shortened. It is a significant effort to use the arm and wrist normally. It takes concerted effort to rebuild the muscles and tendons and remobilize the joints.

When muscles aren't used, some of the muscle cells actually die. As muscle cells die, they are replaced by scar tissue. Less muscle cells mean less strength. Remember, scar tissue involves randomly laid down fibers which do a poor job of bearing loads under stress. The muscle becomes physically smaller, weaker and doesn't act like normal muscle. Given enough time the process of atrophy can result in a muscle that is significantly replaced by scar tissue.

It is fairly common to see muscle atrophy as a result of immobilization of a joint. One of my patients had to have her ankle joint operated on due to a crush injury that almost caused her to lose her foot. Unfortunately, post-surgical trauma and infection caused the joint to fuse. The calf muscles normally move the foot up and down. After her ankle fused and no movement was possible, the calf muscles became much smaller than those of the other leg and the tendons tightened. The calf muscles lost most of their muscle cells and became *fibrotic*. I have seen the same thing in people who had to wear a foot drop brace because nerve damage made it impossible for them to lift their foot or toes.

CONNECTIVE TISSUE MISUSE

Like muscle, the connective tissues of our body are affected by overuse, misuse and abuse. Overstretching our tendons, ligaments and joint capsules can result in tearing. The stretching can be intentional or accidental. The tearing can be large, like a third-degree strain or a tendon rupture. It can also be microscopic with no obvious signs except for pain and somewhat increased laxity.

One of the most common experiences is tendinitis of the lateral or outside part of the elbow. It is made worse any time you try to use your hand or wrist. It mostly comes from overuse of the wrist, particularly if the motion involves twisting the wrist or a repetitive flexion and extension of the wrist while twisting the forearm. Since these are the descriptions of the motions in tennis, it is generally referred to as "tennis elbow." The actual injury involves the tendons of the forearm muscles that cause the wrist and fingers to extend away from the palm. These muscles attach to the outside bony extension of the elbow (called the *condyle*). When these muscles are overused, their tendons become inflamed, particularly where they attach to the bone. The tendons are typically swollen, painful, and tender. Probably the fact that the twisting and flexion of the wrist also meets forceful resistance every time the racquet hits the tennis ball contributes. As far as I know there has been no microscopic analysis of these inflamed tendons but microscopic tearing is a good possibility.

A similar situation is seen in the wrist when the hand is used to grip something repetitively. It is made worse if the object being gripped is vibrating. The base of the wrist includes two bones, the *scaphoid* and *lunate*, that form a valley on the palm. The valley is termed the carpal tunnel. This area is filled with connective tissue. In the valley are the arteries that supply blood to the hand and fingers. This connective tissue also contains the nerves that go to the muscles of the hand. These nerves provide sensory input from the hand and fingers and control some of the muscles of the hand and thumb. With repetitive pressure on the carpal tunnel, the connective tissues become inflamed, and this inflammation leads to the development of scar tissue. Eventually the nerves and arteries are compressed. This is carpal tunnel syndrome: numbness, tingling and pain, loss of grip strength and eventual muscle atrophy in the palm muscles of the hand.

CONNECTIVE TISSUE DISUSE

The effect of disuse of a joint can be more subtle than visible atrophy. A common response of any joint that is not moved for more than three or four weeks is that the joint itself stiffens. Its range of motion becomes much more limited and defined by the immobilized position. For instance, a finger that has been splinted for more than 21 days is typically quite difficult to bend for a while after.

The mechanisms behind the stiffening and shortening of connective tissue are relatively simple. Recall that normal use of any connective tissue also maintains its flexibility and the optimal orientation of the fibers along the lines of stress. The cells of the connective tissue and their protein fibers are always turning over. Ongoing normal use causes the new cells and the fibers they produce to be laid down in the same fashion as those they replaced. However, if there is no stress on the tissue the new cells and the fibers they produce are laid down in a random pattern. Immobilized connective tissue rearranges into a random meshwork, much like scar tissue. The tissue is less dense, less flexible, shorter and weak. Under a normal load it is much more easily torn. If this were to occur around the shoulder, for example, it could lead to a frozen shoulder.

INACTIVITY, ATROPHY AND PAIN

Recall that virtually all of the pain receptors are found in the connective tissues. When muscles and tendons atrophy, the normal structures are replaced by atrophic scarring. With this increase in connective tissue there may be more pain receptors. The implication of this is that attempting to use atrophic muscles and tendons activates more pain receptors than if it remains unused. Joint disuse causes reorganization of the fibers in the ligaments and joint capsule. The normally high concentration of pain fiber endings in these structures are more easily activated because the joint structures are no longer structured to handle normal loads and movements. Because of these complementary processes, inactivity leads to pain.

Clearly pain is a strong disincentive to using that part of the body. Using a damaged or broken part of the body typically results in even more damage. Pain protects us from further damage by preventing use. But that very disuse leads to further degeneration.

When pain is severe, but tied to particular activities, we instinctively stop those activities in order to avoid the pain. One of my patients came to my office after an absence of about eight months. About six weeks prior to seeing me he had developed pain in his right shoulder. He denied any injury although he had been playing a lot of tennis prior to developing his shoulder pain. He had stopped playing tennis when the pain started. Years before he had a partial rotator cuff tear in his left shoulder that ultimately required surgery. The new pain in his shoulder was similar but different. For one thing, it was not a particular movement of his shoulder that caused pain. He would have pain even if he lay on it in bed causing him to sleep on his left side or back. In short, any activity that involved moving his shoulder became painful. He tried aspirin, ibuprofen and Tylenol, all without much relief. By the time he came to see me he was showing signs of limited range of motion in his shoulder. My evaluation showed no evidence of rotator cuff tear. He did have some mild grating and popping in his shoulder, but no more than he had in the past. The main thing was that he had tenderness of many of the bursal sacks that surround the shoulder and keep the tendons from rubbing on the bone and vice versa. This bursitis will resolve readily if injected with steroid. Before and after the injection his shoulder was mobilized manually. Because of the pain-blocking effect of the anesthetics that I used, mixed with the steroid injection, he was able to tolerate the pain when I moved it. Since the steroid effect lasted a few days, he continued to move it and so kept it from freezing up again. Within days he had full use of his shoulder.

Obviously, pain can cause us to stop using a body part, even an essential body part, and even knowing what is happening. Contrary to the old saying, "use it or lose it," pain can be bad enough to prevent use. When that happens, muscle and connective tissue atrophy and joint capsule reorganization can set in, completing a process that leads to immobilization.

The disuse-atrophy-pain-disuse cycle will reinforce changes in the tissues themselves due to inappropriate use or disuse. The disuse-atrophy cycle can make the recovery from skeletal immobilization quite a painful process. One example in my practice was a 41-year-old woman who had breast cancer. A right hander, she had a left mastectomy which left her chest wall muscles intact and sentinel node biopsy because the tumor had been about 1 ½ inches. Subsequently she went through a planned breast reduction on the right side and implant reconstruction on the left side. All in all, her bout with cancer and its aftermath had been quite successful. However, because of the pain of two separate surgeries involving the left chest wall, she had pain in her left shoulder as she attempted to use her arm. Even though she was referred to physical therapy multiple times for mobilization of that shoulder, the pain kept her from using it. Eventually she developed a frozen left shoulder. She could not use that arm even to put her bra on. To put on a blouse or shirt required slipping the left arm through the sleeve first and then awkwardly maneuvering into the garment using only her right arm. Washing her hair could be done only with the right arm and hand. She was even sent to an orthopedic surgeon who performed what is called manipulation under anesthesia. While the patient is under the influence of general anesthesia, the surgeon moves the joint through much of its natural range of motion based on the surgeon's knowledge of joint mechanics. Having performed a couple of these manipulations under anesthesia, I can tell you that tissue resistance is relatively easily overcome when the patient is unable to feel pain and the muscles are relaxed. Unfortunately, the pain after the procedure was so severe that she was unable to use the arm at all. As a result, it froze again. By the time she came to me two years after the surgery she was extremely frustrated. She wanted answers and was willing to try anything.

She carried her left shoulder stiffly at her side. Although she could bend her left elbow, she could not lift her arm forward or to the side more than 20 degrees. The pectoral muscles and those around the scapula as well as the cap of her shoulder (deltoids) were about half the size of the right.

Attempts to passively raise her arm to the front or side or to bring it backward or across the front of her body gave her a few extra degrees of motion, but beyond that a sharp and severe pain.

After clearly identifying her range of motion limits and being sure that there were no tears or arthritic impingements in her left shoulder, I set up a program to help her regain its use. The model I used involved focusing on one range of motion limitation at a time. Part of that program involved manual manipulative treatment to her neck, upper back and left shoulder every two weeks. With the shoulder I would work with all limitations. However, I would focus on one. The patient's role in this program was not passive. Fortunately, she was quite willing to do the daily home exercise and stretching needed. Based on my experiences I knew that each one of the necessary exercises would be painful, particularly when it was first introduced. I limited her to one new exercise/stretch routine aimed at a particular set of muscles at a time. When she had mastered that one and restored that range of motion to at least 80% of normal, I would add the next. After about four months, her left shoulder had recovered about 90% of its normal range and use and was largely pain free. It has remained normal since.

It is well documented in medical literature that rare individuals are born with a genetic glitch that prevents them from experiencing pain. They can have bad sprains and suffer wounds and feel nothing. They can even break bones without being aware of it. Because they feel nothing, they will continue to use the injured body part. This increases the damage. Most of these individuals live a fairly short life and are often crippled by the badly healed injuries they have suffered without knowing it.

TISSUE STIFFNESS

Stiffness in some parts of the body is almost as common a complaint as pain. Frequently these two complaints go together. It is a common and valid belief that failure to properly stretch before or after exercise can cause stiffness in our connective tissues including joints, tendons, and ligaments. When we stop using a body part due to pain, stiffness is the normal response, followed later by inability to move the part. Presumably this is in part due to the reorganization of connective tissues when they are not subjected to normal stresses. Older people also will tell you that, in general, their joints, tendons, and muscles are stiffer than when they were young.

A partial explanation could be the reorganization of the tissues with more random and less organized connective tissue due to periodic disuse and the accumulation of small traumas.

There is a particular case of tissue stiffness found in some diabetics. When a person's blood sugar remains high for more than a month or two, we see sugar molecules binding to proteins throughout the body. The process is termed *glycosylation*. In fact, we use the amount of glucose-bound hemoglobin protein to measure how well a diabetic's blood sugar has been controlled over the preceding three months (*glycosylated hemoglobin or HgbA1c*). When there is significant glucose binding to the hemoglobin molecules the red blood cells become stiff and have a hard time making it through the smallest blood vessels, the capillaries. This produces problems with circulation. It is important to realize that all proteins can become glucose bound. Typically, when they do the long collagen proteins of our tendons, ligaments, and joint capsules become stiffer and more prone to tearing and rupture. This means that uncontrolled diabetes can result in stiffer and more fragile connective tissues including those of the joint, muscles, tendons, and ligaments.

TISSUE LAXITY AFTER INJURY

In rare cases, the damage to supporting tissues around a joint or muscle is so extreme that even after the tissues heal there is still laxity in those tissues. This is often the case in second-degree ankle sprains where there has been some tearing in the ligaments and tendons supporting the ankle, but not complete tearing that would require surgery. I've also seen this kind of laxity in shoulders that have been repeatedly dislocated. It is also fairly common in the joint between the sacrum and the pelvis bones after being repeatedly "treated" with a lot of force. In each case there is too much motion and no stability. I also see it frequently in people who "crack" their neck or back multiple times a day.

Because of the laxity in the joint, muscle, or ligament, it is more difficult to use it properly. In some cases, one can build extra muscle strength around the lax tissue. Because of the laxity the tissue is subject to additional and repeated injury. For instance, a knee with a lax ligament may be too unstable to allow the person to stand and walk on that leg. We have few options in such a case. We need to do something to shorten and strengthen the tissue. This can be done by injections that cause tissue tightening (*prolotherapy* or platelet-rich plasma), surgery or wearing a brace or other device that immobilizes the joint or lax tissue.

HYPERMOBILITY SYNDROMES

Some of the most remarkable and persistent problems with body pain I have encountered are in people who appear to have genetically based tissue laxity, or hypermobility syndrome. Many of these patients reported having been double-jointed when they were young. They could bend their thumb back to touch their wrist. They could do splits easily. Often, they could bring their ankle up and behind their head. They also typically report that others in their family were similarly double-jointed. They don't seem to be aware of other problems related to their connective tissue laxity although sometimes they may also demonstrate a heart valve click or murmur.

It would seem as though people with hypermobility syndrome are blessed. They don't have the stiffness in muscles and joints that many of the rest of us have. In fact, many are involved in athletic activities that emphasize flexibility, such as gymnastics, yoga, or dance.

Unfortunately, many people with hypermobility syndrome are addicted to stretching. They routinely stretch their muscles, tendons, ligaments, and joints to the limit of what is anatomically allowed. While this may seem like a good thing, in fact it is not. If the tissue is already stretched to its maximum and a traumatic force is introduced, the muscle, tendon, ligament, or joint may be carried beyond its ability to function, creating instability and pain. The other complication that seems to arise frequently in people who have hypermobility syndrome is the development of early and sometimes severe osteoarthritis, presumably due to repetitive injuries.

One woman has been my patient now for a long time. Her first presentation for body pain came after she had repeatedly driven a car with a broken seat while doing route sales. It had not occurred to her that the broken seat might cause a problem. Eventually she developed a chronic pain in her lower back and hip even when she was not in the car. That pain would persist even when she was on vacation and not driving at all. When she came to see me, she had an upward shear of her pelvis on one side. After appropriate manual treatment she would leave the office balanced and pain free. However, she would have the same hip sheared upward by the next time she came in for treatment. It took me several visits and persistent questioning to realize that her car seat was the apparent source of her returning pain. She did get the car seat repaired. I expected, based on my experience with other people who had similar problems, that the upward shear of her pelvis would rapidly resolve. It did not. It took almost 10 more treatments over a period of three months before she came back with no pain and no pelvic shear.

Over the next few years, I would see her back again many times. Sometimes it was from lifting something wrong, or from a fall. One time it was a minor motor vehicle accident. Each time it took many more treatments to get her problems to resolve than would have been the case for others. Finally, she tripped and fell, producing a moderate foot and ankle strain. There was no apparent tearing of the tissues and no bone fracture, but the recovery was long and stormy.

At that point I began to suspect that she had some problem with her connective tissues. She admitted on questioning that she had been double-jointed as a child. She was still quite flexible even in her 40s. She could still bend her thumb back and touch it to her wrist. She also was addicted to stretching, partly because it felt so good and partly because she had always been told that stretching was what she should do for painful muscles and tendons. On questioning, her sister was having similar problems. Suspecting she might have one of the connective tissue diseases known to cause hypermobility, I had a tissue biopsy performed. All of her lab and pathology results were normal. As in all of her previous problems, healing from her surgery was slow and rocky. In recent years she has developed early osteoarthritis in her spine, hips, and knees.

Most people with hypermobility syndrome do not have any clear tissue pathology nor do they have any laboratory findings that can conclusively give us a diagnosis. The assumption is that some components of the connective tissue are just a little different from normal. What is clear is that these people have a major problem with muscle, tendon, ligament, and joint healing in addition to their hypermobility. Over the years since I first began seeing this patient, I have found others who present in the same fashion with greatly prolonged body healing. I can only assume that this is a standard problem for people with this condition.

The only strategy I have found that helps people with hypermobility syndrome is for them to get involved in a daily strenuous exercise program that does not involve any stretching. And, when they come back with body pain, to make sure they do so as soon as it develops. Having stronger muscles and not stretching seems to improve their ability to hold normal functional relationships in their body without having to be treated all the time. This advice is the exact opposite of the integration of stretching with muscle strengthening that we recommend for people who don't have hypermobility syndrome.

Sometimes hypermobility syndrome is a part of a genetic disease called Ehlers-Danlos syndrome. There are actually multiple diseases that are grouped under the name Ehlers-Danlos. Many of these diseases are discovered in childhood and involve such severe derangements of connective tissue function that many do not survive childhood. Some have laxity of skin, heart valves, eye structures, and blood vessels in addition to joint capsules, tendons, and ligaments. One subgroup is termed Ehlers-Danlos type 1. Although Ehlers-Danlos type 1 may be discovered in childhood, for the most part it is a fairly benign disease that is discovered in adulthood. It looks like the hypermobility syndrome described above. The only way to demonstrate that hypermobility is in fact Ehlers-Danlos type 1 is by examining some of the connective tissue in a specialized pathology laboratory. It may be the case that some of those who have been diagnosed with hypermobility syndrome have Ehlers-Danlos type 1. For the most part, treatment of Ehlers-Danlos type 1 is similar to that described for general hypermobility syndrome.

The other genetic hypermobility syndrome that bears some comment is Marfan syndrome. In this connective tissue disease, the patients are typically tall and slender. Their limbs, fingers, and toes are unusually long. They have excessive flexibility of their joints. They may have instability in their major arteries coming from the heart including development of aneurisms. Many have flattened or even caved in front chest walls termed *pectus excavatum*.

CHAPTER 5
The Nature of Pain

Even though most of my patients come to me with muscle, tendon, ligament, and joint restrictions and a decrease in normal functioning, frequently it is the accompanying pain that brings them through my doors. In previous chapters we discussed some of the roles that pain plays in injury and healing. So, what is pain?

Pain is an experience, a trigger for behavior, and a cause of emotion. Pain is essentially a signal in the brain, spinal cord and nerves that something damaging is happening to the body. It can be sharp, immediate, demanding, in your face. It can be sharply focused and well localized. However, pain can also be spread out, indistinct, covering a broad area of the body, or even moving from place to place. It can be dull, grinding, and persistent and worm its way into your life and consciousness. Either way, whether it is very intense or just persistent, it can become a major focus of your life – even dominating your life. It often affects sleep, personal and work relationships, and sex life. It may stop a person from working, or even from performing the normal activities of daily living.

The Oxford dictionary definition of pain is "a range of unpleasant bodily sensations produced by illness, accident, etc." It is difficult to describe in words exactly what pain is, though we certainly know it when we feel it. In English we tend to describe pain in terms of an analogy. Pain is "sharp and piercing" or "stabbing" because at times it is like we have been stabbed by a sharp object. Pain can be "crushing" when it feels like a body part being crushed by a heavy weight or being pressed between two hard objects. Pain can be described as "burning" or "searing." Sometimes we are reduced to describing pain in terms of what else is happening at the same time. Thus, pain is sometimes described as cramping, spasming, or writhing.

TYPES OF PAIN

Scientists and doctors have tended to divide pain into two different types based on its source and how it presents itself. *Epicritic pain* is sharp, intense, and highly focused in its location. The tendency is to identify this type of pain with skin and musculoskeletal origins. *Protopathic pain* is more dull, diffuse and hard to localize. This type of pain is said to be from the internal organs of the body, the viscera. Similarly, epicritic pain pathways are said to be more similar to those from other skin sensations, like touch. Protopathic pain supposedly involves more primitive pain pathways. Protopathic pain is proposed to be more likely to involve emotional states. Epicritic pain is not.

Unfortunately, in my experience and that of most of my patients, the identification of muscle, tendon, ligament, joint, and bone pain as being largely epicritic is not very accurate. Actual muscle, tendon, and joint pain can share both sharpness and diffuseness at the same time and from the same source. It can even alternate from being sharp and intense at times to being dull and spread out at other times. Whether sharply localized or quite diffuse, pain can range from very minimal to quite intense. It can be quite brief or persistent, lasting for years. It can be intermittent or constant. Clearly the scientific categories of epicritic and protopathic pain have qualities that simultaneously can be found in the spectrum of muscle, tendon, ligament, joint, and bone pain.

ANATOMY OF PAIN

The anatomy of pain is quite complex. To understand it at the level of a physician who specializes in pain would involve a whole book on that single topic. However, there are a number of important facts about the anatomy and physiology underlying pain that will help us understand pain and its management. Pain usually starts with tissue that is injured enough to trigger a particular type of sensory nerve cell called a *nociceptor*. When triggered, the pain nerve endings do two things. First, they release local chemicals into the tissue. Some of these chemicals signal the immune system and start a healing response, while other chemicals produce a local response that increases blood flow to the tissue, local swelling and inflammation. Second, the free nerve endings trigger transmission of a signal that travels along wire-like microscopic fibers toward the nociceptor cell body and ultimately to the spinal cord and brain.

PAIN IS IN THE BRAIN

In reality, unless that pain signal reaches the brain, and particularly the part of the brain called the cerebral cortex, there is no experience of pain.

There can be tissue reactions to damaging or potentially damaging events and there can be reflex events as the body tries to avoid further damage. Truly though, pain resides in the brain.

Unless the information from the body gets to the cerebral cortex, there is no pain. The cerebral cortex lies just inside much of our skull. It more or less sits at the top of the complex organ termed the central nervous system (Fig. 5-1a). The cortex is far larger in humans than in most other animals. It is commonly held that the cortex is the center of consciousness, although this is probably an over-simplification. The structure of the cerebral cortex is quite complex, but basically it receives and processes sensory inputs, builds memory, correlates sensory information with memory, other senses and emotions, and directs voluntary action.

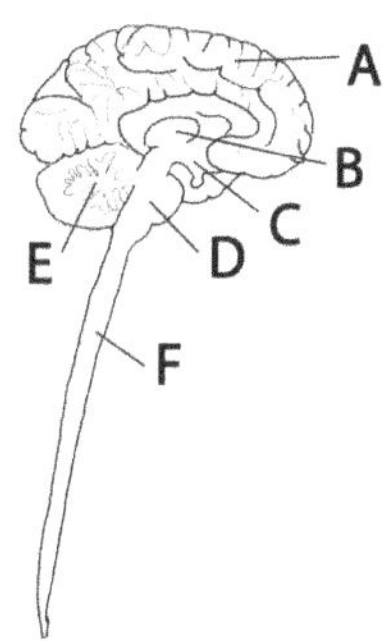

When parts of the cerebral cortex are damaged as a result of a stroke or surgery, we may lose voluntary control of parts of the body (paralysis). For instance, if there is damage to a part of the right lateral cortex, we may lose control of the left leg and arm. We might also lose sensation and awareness of the left leg and arm depending on how much of the cortex is damaged. In this case, where there is no awareness of sensations from the left leg and arm, there may be no pain. Literally, we may become permanently anesthetized for that part of the body.

There are many other circumstances in which potentially painful inputs do not reach the cerebral cortex and therefore the pain is not experienced. Most of them have to do with what is loosely termed attention. There are multiple instances in which attention can be both the source of pain perception and block that perception.

First, most of us have experiences in which a painful stimulus is so strong and demanding that we can literally think of nothing else. It feels to us as if the pain itself is grabbing our attention. It won't let us focus on anything else. It so dominates our life that we may fail to perform basic activities of daily living such as eating or sleeping, performing basic acts of hygiene like bathing, or combing our hair. Our social and work obligations may be performed poorly or not at all. All we can focus on is the pain itself and our attempts to make it go away. Fortunately for most of us, this hyperfocus on pain may be only temporary. In other instances, it persists and becomes the defining aspect of someone's life. In either case, the pain becomes so dominant because our attention is focused on it.

We all have experiences in which we just ignore pain or do something else hoping we can make pain recede into the background. That stimulus, which in other circumstances would be experienced as painful, becomes much less so. Sometimes that is because we "will" it to be less. We all know about the Indian Yogis who appear to be able to block significant pain even from something as serious as a knife wound. More often, we find something else to do that captures our attention. As we do that something else, the pain may be forgotten, at least for a while. Whether that is something physical, such as swimming, or painting, or a mental activity, like being absorbed in a good book, or a conversation, the pain decreases and moves into the background. It may even temporarily disappear.

The brain mechanisms that drive our ability to focus on something start in the brainstem but are largely dependent on the thalamus and cerebral cortex. The thalamus is a processing center just below the cortex (Fig. 5-1b). Anatomically it is buried inside the cerebral cortex. Virtually all information coming to and leaving the cortex goes through the thalamus. Whether it is because of a flood of information from another sense or simply as a result of our attending to another task, pain can be blocked. On the other hand, when pain captures our attention, we may not be able to do even the most basic of tasks. When the thalamus and cerebral cortex are focused on pain, little else exists.

The meaning of pain and its significance in our lives is also the result of the pain signal reaching the cerebral cortex and being processed there. Pain as an immediate experience is something that we try to avoid. However, we also can have a lot of learned associations with pain. We can learn that pain can be rewarded and thus sought out. We may learn to associate pain and pleasure. We may be so afraid of some type of pain, like cancer or a heart attack, that every painful event becomes the signal that cancer is present or a heart attack is occurring. These learned associations occur in the cerebral cortex. Cortex damage can make them better or worse depending on what is damaged.

THE NEURAL CONNECTION BETWEEN EMOTION AND PAIN

The hypothalamus lies at the bottom of the brain in the center under the thalamus (Fig. 5-1c). It is intimately involved in sexuality, hunger, and other appetites, our emotions, and our sense of smell. Along with the thalamus and cortex, the hypothalamus also receives pain-related inputs. When a pain signal reaches the hypothalamus from the spinal cord or brainstem, it triggers an emotional response, particularly those we term negative, like fear, anger, anxiety, and depression.

The physical expression of emotion comes from the output of the hypothalamus to the brainstem and spinal cord (Fig 5-1d,f). Part of this involves controlling the sympathetic nervous system, as we shall see below. Pupils enlarge or become pinpoint, skin flushes, the heart races or slows down, reaction times speed up or slow down, physical activity increases or decreases, all under the direction of the emotion centers in the hypothalamus.

The hypothalamus also is connected to the cerebral cortex. Thus, the meaning of the emotion states and the relationship between emotions, pain and learning all come about because the hypothalamus sends its messages forward to the thalamus and cerebral cortex.

Likewise, part of the modulation of pain involves the generation of a type of chemical transmitter called the endorphins. The endorphins are either produced by the hypothalamus and released into the blood stream or produced by neurons that originate in the hypothalamus and go to other parts of the upper nervous system, brainstem and spinal cord.

The endorphins are part of a system than helps modulate and, in some cases, block pain. They produce virtually the same response as opiates such as morphine, heroin, cocaine, oxycodone, and hydrocodone. Opiates are all either naturally occurring chemicals from plants or man-made versions. All block pain, both at the nociceptor, and at multiple points in the spinal cord, brainstem and brain. They also produce euphoria, and can produce delusional states, nausea, and constipation. The story of the discovery of the endorphins is a fascinating part of the development of modern neurochemistry. However, it is sufficient to our current discussion to know that the endorphins originate within the hypothalamus and are related to both emotional states and pain control.

THE SYMPATHETIC NERVOUS SYSTEM

Recall that pain usually starts with tissue that is injured enough to trigger a particular type of sensory nerve cell called a nociceptor. The sensing end of pain receptors are embedded in connective tissue everywhere in the body except in the brain itself. Most nociceptors send their fibers within very fine nerves that travel with blood vessels. The cell bodies for these pain receptors are clustered together in the sympathetic ganglia. The sympathetic ganglia are part of the autonomic nervous system, which exists outside of the brain or along the spinal column. The importance of this is not readily apparent until we understand what the autonomic nervous system is.

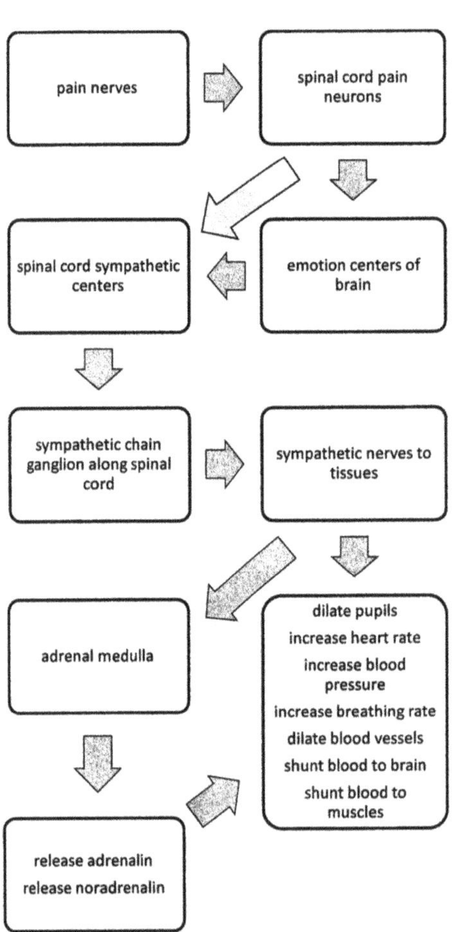

The autonomic nervous system is the management system that balances normal healthy functioning in most of our internal organs. It also helps produce responses to threats and potentially damaging events. It is largely involuntary, though not unconscious. We are aware of its function at some level throughout our lives.

Half of the autonomic nervous system basically keeps our organs running at an interactive functional level. This is the *parasympathetic nervous system*. It keeps the gut processing food, the blood flow to the gut picking up nutrients and delivering them to the rest of the body, our saliva flowing, and sweat glands operating to help control body temperature. It diverts blood from the muscles to the gut and keeps blood flowing to the kidneys. It lowers blood pressure and keeps our heart rate stable. It slows and calms breathing.

The other half of the autonomic nervous system, termed the *sympathetic nervous system,* is the critical actor in relation to pain (Fig. 5-2). Remember that the cell bodies for pain nerves are mostly found in the sympathetic ganglia. These ganglia are lined up on either side of the spine behind the chest and part of the abdomen. The sympathetic cell bodies in the ganglia produce nerve fibers that go out to and control blood vessels, the heart, lungs and most other organs using a neurotransmitter called epinephrine. The sympathetic nervous system also connects to the inside part of two glands that sit on top of each kidney, the adrenal glands. The *adrenal medulla* ("middle") produces adrenaline and noradrenalin when it is stimulated by the sympathetic nerves. These chemicals enter the bloodstream where they reinforce the effect of the sympathetic nerves on blood vessels and other organs.

Functionally, the sympathetic nervous system shunts blood to the brain and skeletal muscles and away from the gut. It increases heart rate, blood pressure and the breathing rate. It causes the pupils of the eyes to dilate. It dilates blood vessels in the skin. It causes our hairs to stand on end. Its activation is experienced as the fright, fight or flight response.

One of the big triggers for the sympathetic nervous system is pain and the threat of injury. Remember that the pain receptors have their cell bodies in the sympathetic ganglia. This provides for a very quick pathway for a pain stimulus to activate the sympathetic nervous system.

Pain receptor fibers also travel in nerves to the spinal cord and brain where they terminate in other neurons. Some of these neurons then feed back onto pre-motor neurons that feed back to the sympathetic chain ganglia and produce an additional amplification and widening of the sympathetic response to pain.

Many of the emotion centers in the upper brain send signals down to the spinal cord and out to the sympathetic ganglia. When the emotion centers of the upper brain are triggered by painful inputs, they feed back on the sympathetic ganglia. This further amplifies the sympathetic response to pain.

Finally, it should be noted that both the adrenalin and noradrenalin produced by the adrenal medulla and dumped into the blood seem to amplify the pain signal coming from pain receptors. Additionally, the sympathetic nerves produce epinephrine, which is chemically almost identical to adrenalin at their nerve endings. Since many sympathetic nerve endings are found in the same tissues where we find the pain receptors, similar amplification of pain signals can occur.

What does all of this mean? There is a tight relationship between the pain pathways and the sympathetic nervous system. Events that trigger the pain receptors are quite likely to also trigger the body responses that lead to fright, flight or fight. At the same time, the sympathetic responses tend to amplify the painful inputs, making them even worse.

EDITING PAIN IN THE BRAINSTEM AND SPINAL CORD

Remembering that many pain nerves have their cell bodies in the sympathetic ganglia, these pain nerves or nociceptors send fibers into the spinal cord (buried inside the spine) or brainstem (at the base of the brain). Other pain receptors have their cell bodies in ganglia along with touch sensation nerves. These often allow us to better localize the site of injury. However, both types of pain receptors send fibers into the spinal cord and brainstem.

In the spinal cord and brainstem, these pain receptors terminate (synapse) on other neurons that will process the information. Many of these secondary neurons are local, staying at or near the level where the pain nerves entered. Some of these local neurons contact the motor neurons that produce pain reflexes and stimulate the sympathetic response. Others are involved in a form of feed-forward messaging that can amplify the signal coming in from the pain receptors. Particularly when there are many pain receptors reporting at the same time, there may actually be a ramping up of the pain signal, ensuring that the signal gets through to higher centers.

Some local spinal neurons are involved in a form of feedback that can modulate and sometimes even block the pain signals. For instance, if there is a strong touch stimulus in an area of the body near the site of pain, the pain may be less intense or may not be sensed at all. The touch sensors apparently stimulate some local neurons in the spinal cord that then block the pain signals. This is the basis for the use of many of today's electrical stimulators, such as the TENS units, and some of the spinal cord stimulators used to block pain in chronic pain patients.

Some of the spinal cord and brainstem pain-related neurons send their fibers on up toward the brain. Some of these long-distance fibers go to an area in the brainstem termed the *periaqueductal gray*. This is an ancient structure found in the nervous system of all animals with vertebrae. It is part of the attention and arousal system. It also feeds back on the lower pathways that go to the sympathetic nervous system to amplify any response.

The remainder of the long-distance pain pathways go to the thalamus and after that to the cortex or to the hypothalamus and then the cortex. Pathways from the hypothalamus and thalamus as well as the cerebral cortex also descend to the brainstem and spinal cord where they can affect both the pain sensory input, the touch sensory input, and the motor outputs to muscles and the sympathetic nervous system.

Thus, each level of the nervous system can feed back to either amplify or block the pain signal coming from damaged tissue. One of the basic truths about pain is that it is not always what it seems to be. As we shall see, while pain may be felt in a particular area of the body, there can be potentially painful stimuli other places, as well. The same pain stimulus may present as pain at one time and not felt at other times. A painful stimulus may be present but not felt. But when another painful stimulus is added, like the proverbial straw that broke the camel's back, the pain may suddenly be outrageous.

CHAPTER 6
Pain is Liar

Years ago, when I was in my internship, I was seeing a 40-year-old patient with my mentor, Dr. Dzmura. The patient was complaining about pain in his left neck and shoulder. He was quite calm and denied feeling short of breath or experiencing pressure on his chest. Dr. Dzmura asked me what I thought we should do. I said I thought we should listen to his heart and lungs, check his blood pressure, give him a nitroglycerin tablet and do an EKG to check his heart. I also thought that perhaps we should call an ambulance to take him to the hospital. When the initial cardiac and lung evaluation proved to be normal and the nitroglycerin had no effect on the patient's pain, Dr. Dzmura asked whether I still thought we should call the ambulance. He pointed out that I had not asked the patient anything about the circumstances of this pain, including whether he had eaten anything that might cause heartburn, had fallen or done anything that might have injured his neck, shoulder, arm or chest, and whether there was anything that would make the pain less or worse. Ashamed that I had jumped to conclusions without fully evaluating the patient, I set to work.

Later, after completing the patient's workup we were able to relieve his pain with musculoskeletal manipulation. We did determine that he should see a cardiologist for further evaluation because he had a family history of early cardiac disease. However, there was no cardiac emergency.

After the patient left, Dr. Dzmura took me into his office and gave me a concept that is central to my diagnostic world view. He said, "Pain is a liar." Then he went on to explain. In this case, pain could have represented something wrong with the heart, the esophagus or the neck and shoulder. In fact, pain in many of the internal organs can present as pain in some part of the musculoskeletal system. As we have seen in a number of cases previously, pain in one part of the musculoskeletal system can be caused by structural or functional injuries in other parts of the body. In some cases, pain can seem to wander around in the soma because, in fact, many parts are potentially painful but the brain sees only the part that is yelling the loudest at the moment. An injury that would be painful for most people can potentially cause no pain.

Pain can exist where there was injury in the past and, even though it has healed, there is still pain. Pain can exist even where there is no structural or functional imbalance. And finally, as is seen in the phenomenon call phantom limb pain, pain can be felt even in a body part that no longer is present.

All these phenomena mean for the physician that pain is a signal that something needs to be evaluated and hopefully diagnosed and treated. It tells us something is wrong, but not necessarily what. The reason that pain is potentially disconnected to actual injury is that the experience of pain is actually in the brain. If the brain misinterprets the pain signals, the experience will be different from reality.

PAIN = DAMAGE

Pain is almost always taken by the person experiencing it as signaling damage that may be occurring in or to the body. The damage may be quite real and serious. At other times, however, the pain may only be a response to the potential for damage. The body is telling us that if we continue with what we have been doing we will suffer damage. Sometimes pain tells us that damage has occurred in the past. In all cases, whether damage is present or not, pain is interpreted in the same way: that injury is present.

It is easy to see why there is pain when there is a fresh burn on the skin, or a broken bone, or someone has a recent surgery site that hasn't yet healed. As a side note, we should keep in mind that any surgery involves not only cutting through the skin, but also the cutting and disruption of muscle and connective tissue and sometimes even bone. We expect pain if we have a bruise or a torn muscle or ruptured tendon. In every case, the actual damage to our tissue yields pain.

The pain comes from the nociceptor nerve endings that are within and at the margins of the damaged tissue. These specialized pain nerves generate a series of local and whole-body responses that should keep us from further harm and help promote healing. The experience of pain is a necessary part of these responses.

Although we do not like the experience, pain prevents us from doing something that might further injure the already damaged tissue. The pain itself acts to rein in activity that could keep the tissue from healing. And, as we discussed briefly before, pain actually plays a role in the healing process itself. If we later over-exert ourselves, we will develop muscle pain. The muscle needs time to recover from our exertions, and pain will force us to limit our use of that muscle for a while.

Similarly, if we do something that might cause damage but hasn't yet done so, the body may generate a pain signal to prevent us from going further and actually injuring ourselves. We see this kind of response when we slightly overstretch a muscle, tendon, or a joint. Presumably this painful stimulus occurs because of microscopic tissue injury. The actual damage is minimal, but the pain signal keeps us from stretching the damaged tissue any further. Thus, stressing our tissues can cause pain even where there is little actual damage.

In other cases, pain tells us that damage has occurred in the past. For example, if a scar has left the skin tight and distorted, it is easy to see that any activity that might stretch the scar may provoke pain. If a bone has been broken and heals with an abnormal shape or size, it is easy to see how its changed ability to function might cause pain.

Consider the case of my great aunt who suffered multiple fractures of her pelvis and one leg as a child when a horse she was riding fell on her. When her injuries finally healed, one leg was 8 inches shorter than the other. For the rest of her life, she wore a prosthetic shoe that added about 6 inches to the shortened leg. In response, she developed a severe scoliosis (sideways bending of her spine). In this case, the damage left the musculoskeletal system distorted and dysfunctional. It would be a wonder if she didn't have chronic pain. Unfortunately, if she was to walk or even sit, she was going to have pain. In a sense her pain was from both the past injuries and from the terrible compromises her body had to make for her to stand upright and walk. Her musculoskeletal system was always under stress. The pain stimulus was there to keep her from doing any further damage. Unfortunately, the damage had already been done long ago.

Most of my patients do not have anything quite so obvious. For example, if they had a broken bone or a sprain, the bone or joint is now well healed without any sign of infection or obvious inflammation. Surgical implants, such as artificial hips or knees, have healed to the surgeon's satisfaction. If they had some other surgery, the tissue is well healed. In fact, the initiating trauma might or might not even be remembered. The signs of what's left behind are often very subtle. Indeed, in most cases X-rays, CT-scans or MRIs show nothing particularly out of the ordinary. But still, the pain is present.

PAIN AND INFLAMMATION

Commonly, pain and inflammation are present at the same time. In fact, many of the medications used to treat inflammation also decrease pain. The reason is actually fairly simple. Remember from our previous discussion that inflammation occurs whenever tissue is damaged. It is part of the mechanism that will lead to healing. Inflammation involves the release of a complex stew of chemicals into damaged tissue. The chemicals are released by the damaged cells, by the nerves in the neighborhood, and by the inflammatory cells that are attracted to the area by the chemical stew. The inflammatory cells include those that will ultimately repair the damage. Key ingredients in this chemical stew include the *prostaglandins* and inflammatory *cytokines*. A number of these chemicals tend to stimulate pain nerve endings in the area, producing pain signals that ultimately end up in the spinal cord and brain.

PAIN IS A GOVERNOR OF OUR ACTIONS

When pain acts as a governor of our actions, it is acting as a trigger for behavior. Sometimes the behavior is one of disuse. Sometimes it is a more subtle change in how we do something to minimize further pain. A classic example of pain acting as a governor is the withdrawal reflex that we discussed earlier. If we touch an object that is hot enough to burn our skin, the automatic response is to pull away. If a dog gets a thorn in its paw, it will pull the leg up and walk on three legs. Although we might see this behavior as a voluntary act, it is, in fact, a very basic nervous system connection directly from the pain receptor to the muscle. This is a behavior that occurs without conscious thought or intent. The withdrawal reflex is unconsciously preventing further pain.

Like the dog or the person unintentionally playing with fire, most pain acts as a stimulus to avoid. Pain has such negative impact that we will significantly change our behavior to avoid it and whatever is causing it. Often when pain first develops in a part of the musculoskeletal system our response is to think something is torn or broken. We all know that the proper response to a broken bone is to immobilize it. In fact, immobilizing it both decreases the pain and gives the bone a better chance to heal. The normal prescription for broken bones and torn tendons is about six weeks of disuse generally accompanied by splinting or casting. We would probably disrupt the healing mechanisms if we were to actually use the broken or torn part.

This idea that a broken or torn part shouldn't be used is so strongly ingrained that it frequently gets in the way of proper recovery. One example is what happens with a muscle tear. Consider the case of a patient in my practice. She was a 50-year-old avid tennis player. Fortunately, she knows to stretch before she plays and has rarely suffered injuries on the tennis court. One time, however, she was on an extended vacation. She went out later in the day to play a little pick-up game of doubles. She felt that because she had stretched first thing in the morning, she would not need to do any further stretching. During the game she bent to hit a low ball, only to have it returned fast and high. She jumped and swung. While she successfully returned the ball, as she came down, she was off-balance and unprepared. She landed with her right knee slightly flexed and all her body weight on it. She fell, rapidly flexing the right knee to its maximum. Fortunately, she did not damage the knee itself. However, she felt an immediate stinging in the front of her right thigh. This rapidly became swollen and painful enough that she had a hard time walking on it. By that evening she saw clear bruising. She put ice on it and went to see a local orthopedic surgeon the next day. He examined her hip, thigh, and knee. After X-rays and a physical examination confirmed there was no significant damage to either her hip or knee joint, he told her that she had torn part of her quadriceps muscle. He advised her to minimize walking, use ice for another day or two and then moist heat. He did not tell her how long she should stay off her leg. She asked a trainer at the local gym, who told her to stay off it for four to six weeks to let it heal. Unfortunately, that was the rest of her vacation, which meant that she could do very little. She did use crutches so she could get around. But any time she bent the knee too much or tried walking without the crutches she had pain in her thigh. That in itself was enough to keep her from using her right leg very much.

After returning from her vacation, she came to see me. She was still using one crutch at times. She found it difficult to walk up and down stairs and impossible to play tennis. Likewise, her weekly yoga class and daily stretching had become difficult and painful. She walked with a slight limp. A careful examination showed a palpable gap under the skin signaling a tear in the quadriceps muscle in the middle of the front part of her right thigh. The remaining quadriceps muscle was also quite tight, not allowing her to bend her right knee more than 80 degrees. Her knee was otherwise normal. She had no visible bruising and no sensory problems. She did have some other structural motion asymmetries that responded well to non-traumatic manual medicine techniques. Unfortunately, I had to resort to more painful stretches to break up the scar tissue that had accumulated in the tear. She was taught similar techniques to use at home. Within three weeks she had full normal range of motion in her knee and hip and no more pain.

In the case of a muscle tear, the problem is that the muscle tissue will not grow again in the torn area. Instead, scar tissue accumulates within the void. Scar tissue has more pain fibers in it than does muscle itself. Scar tissue is also less flexible than either muscle or normal connective tissue. However, over time and with use that scar tissue will remodel into a linear form that is more flexible and aligned with the fibers of the muscle. If my patient had begun exercising and stretching the torn muscle within the first week after her injury, the scar tissue would have been replaced more or less as it was formed. Then she would not have had to go through the period of disuse, pain, and restricted mobility.

In many cases we do not in fact know whether an injury has caused something to be broken or torn. The pain is significant or sharp and causes us to stop all activity, even though there is no reason to believe that the trauma was severe enough to actually break or tear something. That inactivity then just reinforces the pain.

Fortunately, or unfortunately, the worry may be that something is broken when it is not. Another of my patients is a 37-year-old male who has a job that keeps him in and out of the car and in meetings for much of his work day. Most evenings and all weekend, he works out at the gym, runs or plays baseball or other outdoor sports. When he developed a sudden pain in the low back after a fall, he worried that he had a spinal fracture. His 79-year-old father had suffered a fall and vertebral fracture two years before and my patient was worried the same thing had happened to him. He rested in bed a few days but every time he got out of bed it was agony. He went to an orthopedic back surgeon who ordered an X-ray and then an MRI of his low back. Neither study showed evidence of a spinal fracture. There was some evidence of a disc compression, but it was more chronic. That should have been enough to get him back to doing his normal activity, particularly when the surgeon told him that he did not have a surgical problem. However, even a course of prescribed physical therapy was not sufficient to get him back to normal. In fact, all the physical therapy did was make his pain a little worse.

He came to see me based on the suggestion of a friend. By that time, he was more than six weeks out from his injury. He was convinced that something major was wrong. His pain was absent when he was lying down. However, it returned whenever he sat up and particularly when he stood or walked. Therefore, for six weeks he had not been physically active nor had he been able to work much. To say that he was frustrated was an understatement. He had always prided himself on being fit and physically strong. Now, he said, he could "see my muscles wasting away."

In my examination it was easy to see what he had done in his fall. He had produced an upward shear at his right sacroiliac joint. With the right half of his pelvis sheared upward, his right leg was about ½ inch short. Among other things, this produced a mild sideways (scoliotic) curve in his low back. Bed rest had caused his muscles to weaken some. More significantly, by limiting his exercise and activity he had prevented normal muscle compensation from developing. Whenever he sat or stood his muscles would go into painful spasms. Fortunately, it was relatively easy to reduce the upward pelvic shear and his decompensation with manual medicine. He immediately was able to sit, stand and walk without pain. Cautioning him that he needed a day or two to give his body a chance to begin healing, I told him to take it easy. Then, when he did restart his exercise, he was to start slow and not expect his body to begin where he left off. When he returned for his follow-up two weeks later, he was still pain free and able to go back to work and exercising daily.

EMOTION, INJURY AND PAIN

When pain is strong enough, persistent or unavoidable, it also tends to cause emotional problems. Pain is so clearly identified with an emotional experience that our definitions of the word pain include "mental suffering or distress" (Oxford Dictionary). Again, the synonyms for pain can include words like anguish, affliction, grief, misery, despair, and torment. The link between pain and emotion is strong throughout our body and nervous system, as well. The emotional brain, what is sometimes termed the "primitive core" of our nervous system, includes much of the circuitry involved in pain. Likewise, all emotions are expressed through the body.

The emotions triggered by pain are rarely good or positive. The most common emotions that grow out of pain are fear, anger, anxiety, depression, and despair. There is some indication that pain is almost always accompanied by emotions, particularly when the pain lasts a long time.

PAIN AND FEAR

It is easy to see how pain can evoke fear and anxiety. Pain is an experience we wish to avoid. It is a common experience in those who have had a significantly painful experience that the very threat of a repeat experience provokes fear and anxiety. One patient had a severe burn on her hip and thigh as a young girl when her dress came into contact with the flame of a gas heater. Now an adult and many years removed from the incident she is still quite afraid of any open flame. Her fear prevented her from marrying a man when she found out he smoked. She also will not go into a kitchen where a gas stove is being used or into a room with lit candles. Even though she was aware that handled properly these flames are not likely to hurt her, her fear and anxiety was overwhelming.

This same fear of the reoccurrence of pain often leads people to avoid specific activities that caused pain in the past. Golf is a popular sport among the retired people I treat daily. Frequently I hear stories similar to this one, shared by one of my patients who is a vigorous 80-year-old man who had routinely played golf at least three times a week since he retired at age 62. When I last saw him, he complained about pain in his low back, left leg and hip. He said that it had started for no apparent reason about four months prior while he was up north. Unfortunately, every time he took a swing with his golf club the pain would "really wind up, too." He had not played golf in four months as a result.

While he was upset that he could not play golf, he was more afraid of the pain. The pain was sharp when he took a swing but would persist for several hours after he stopped swinging the club. Over time the pain had become more common even with walking and he had begun to limit that too. By the time he returned to our area, and I saw him, his weight had begun to creep up. He was walking slowly and even using a cane. He was afraid of the pain he experienced any time he tried to move vigorously. When I examined him, it appeared to me that he had simply sheared one hip upward, unbalancing his gait and the way he stood. I had to order an

X-ray of his spine and hip to convince him that he really had not developed a sudden and severe worsening of his mild arthritis. The X-rays confirmed that there was little change in his back and hips. After a couple of manual medical treatments, he was walking without pain and was finally willing to try playing golf again.

PAIN AND ANGER

Pain can also provoke anger. Anger is considered the other side of the coin of fear. Both emotions can be stimulated when the adrenalin starts to flow. As discussed previously, pain stimulates the release of adrenalin. When pain does not lead to fear, it often provokes anger. The anger can be at the event that led to the injury. Or the anger can be at your own body that has let you down. Such anger is often seen in those who are athletic or perform physical jobs and who have never before suffered a debilitating pain.

PAIN AND DEPRESSION

It is exceedingly common for pain to lead to depression, particularly when pain is severe or chronic. At a minimum, pain often leads to resignation or the sense that there is little that can be done to prevent the pain or restore your life. Many of my patients have come to me as a last resort. Since there are very few doctors practicing as I do, I suspect that there are a lot of people out there who have seen many doctors, psychologists, physical therapists, chiropractors, massage therapists, and other alternative therapists with little improvement in their symptoms. If they have become resigned to pain as their lot in life, they lose the belief that there is anything more they can do. I know that when people with persistent pain come to see me and finally get relief, most seem to regain their enthusiasm for life.

The result of this resignation is often depression. Feelings of helplessness and hopelessness become dominant. The more severe or prolonged the pain, the more likely it will result in clinical depression. Not only is depression itself an emotional pain, but there is clear evidence that depression feeds back on physical pain and makes it worse. The patient is no longer willing to exercise or stretch, two activities that could help diminish pain. Inactivity itself worsens depression. The patient's sleep becomes disturbed. If they sleep too much, they lose muscle tone even faster due to inactivity. If they don't sleep enough, the lack of sleep will diminish the possibility of healing and magnify the pain. Often the chronic pain patient ends up on narcotics that further depresses the nervous system and worsens depression. Pain becomes the dominant tone of their life and no activity is pleasurable.

One of my patients had suffered a broken hip, pelvis and lower leg when a young man. After surgery and a year of recovery he had returned to a highly functional and relatively pain-free life even with an anatomically shortened leg. Years later, he suffered another accident, a fall on the ski slope. Although there was no structural damage from this second accident, he was in chronic pain. Since there was no real change in his musculoskeletal system, the only thing the doctors could do for him was to put him on doses of narcotics to try to control the pain. His life went tumbling down the slopes of pain and despair just as had his body had on the ski slopes.

When he first came to see me, he was chronically sleep deprived because pain would wake him as he moved around in his sleep. The narcotics he was on were relatively short-acting, so after about four hours he would need another dose. If he woke during the middle of the night with pain it might take him several hours before he could return to sleep. During the day the narcotics would dull him mentally and significantly slow his reaction times, only to have him crash into a barrier of pain as they wore off. It appeared to him that physical activity was permanently off limits. In addition to the ever-increasing need for narcotics, he was on muscle relaxers to relieve some of the muscle spasms that accompanied his pain. Even when reading quietly, he was either doped enough that he would have to struggle to retain what he was reading or the pain would become a significant drain on his attention. He was significantly depressed. He felt life was barely worth living.

Although he was on an antidepressant medicine before he came to my practice, it was a low dose and not particularly oriented to dealing with his pain-driven depression. One of the early changes I instituted was to start him on a significant dose of the antidepressant *citalopram* (Celexa). This antidepressant is different from most. It is a molecule that is structurally similar to the medication *tramadol* (Ultram), a drug often termed the non-narcotic narcotic. Although tramadol has significant pain-relieving properties through activation of part of the narcotic receptors in the body, it has minimal addiction potential. Citalopram has similar pain-relieving properties though is considerably weaker. On the other hand, citalopram has significant antidepressant activity at a level comparable to the best of the modern antidepressants. This makes it an ideal antidepressant for those with pain-driven depression.

We were also able to find some answers to his poor sleep. As anyone who has been sleep-deprived for any length of time knows, the lack of sleep not only slows our reaction times and body functions, it also becomes a source of depression in and of itself. When depression is already present, sleep deprivation makes it worse. By improving his sleep, we were able to improve his body's self-healing and his depression. Over time this allowed us to decrease his need for narcotics.

In addition to the medication regime, we restarted physical exercise, which also helped improve both his depression and sleep disturbance. Experience has taught us that exercise is in itself an excellent antidepressant. Recent studies have tended to reinforce this common-sense idea. As is well known, physical exercise also improves sleep.

EMOTIONS CAN MAKE PAIN WORSE

Clearly pain can trigger emotions. Even worse, pain can be made worse by emotions. In some cases, our emotions can even trigger pain where none was present before.

Emotional states can bring on musculoskeletal pain or make it worse. Specifically, negative emotions like anxiety, stress, fear, anger and depression seem able to do this. Recently another patient had a minor surgery. The damage to her tissues was minimal but clearly evident with post-operative swelling and bruising. The first day after surgery there was enough pain to warrant taking a mild narcotic. However, beginning the second day after surgery she had minimal pain and no longer required the pain medication, even though the bruising and swelling looked worse. About four days after the surgery, just as her tissue appeared to be improving, she got a series of very stressful calls from her daughter who was away in college. My patient had not been leading an entirely stress-free life even before the surgery. But who among us has no stress in their life? Unfortunately, these calls from her daughter greatly increased her stress and anxiety levels, in part because there was almost nothing she could do about her daughter's problem except be a good listener. As her stress went up, she redeveloped pain in the area of her recent surgery.

Her recurring pain was not caused by any further damage to the site of her surgery. When she came to see me, her surgery site was clearly healing. The problem was that her stress and anxiety acted as an amplifier for those pain signals still present. After this was explained to her and she had a chance to reflect on her stress and its relation to her pain, the pain again subsided.

Over the years I have seen quite a few patients whose emotional turmoil seems to have brought on musculoskeletal pain or made their pain much worse. Take the case of another male patient. He had long had episodes of low back pain. Most of these episodes were brief, lasting no more than five days. All had been triggered by minor injuries when playing baseball or at work. He worked as a building contractor. He had never had disabling pain, although he had to come see me for treatment on several occasions. His primary care physician had ordered an X-ray of his low back during one episode the previous year. The X-ray showed a minor decrease in the disc spaces between his vertebrae and mild osteoarthritis. Most of the time, however, he was pain free.

When my patient came to see me on this occasion, he had severe disabling low back pain. He could not sleep. He had been unable to work for about 10 days. He denied any injury. In fact, for the week prior to developing low back pain he had not even been to the gym or played ball. His primary care physician had already checked him for abdominal and bladder problems in the off chance that his pain had come from internal organs. After prolonged discussion I began evaluating his back for any signs of motion and position abnormalities or muscle spasms. As I did so he told me that his girlfriend had walked out on him the day before his back pain started. Although they had been fighting for more than a week when she left him, he was shocked, angry and upset. He had already purchased a ring and was planning to ask her to marry him, so the breakup was unexpected. It appeared that the emotional shock and pain had isolated itself in his "weak link," his back. As I treated his back and hips using manual medicine, he talked about how much this breakup had hurt him. His low back pain resolved over the course of the treatment session. His emotional pain took a little longer until he was able to tell his ex-girlfriend how much the breakup had hurt him, both literally and figuratively.

Recently I began to treat another patient who had a long and involved medical history. She had experienced several bouts with different kinds of cancer with the associated surgeries, radiation and chemotherapy. She had at one time been quite successful in business between the bouts with cancer. However, after a few significant bad turns in her business she was broke and about to lose her home. She was severely depressed. She no longer dressed professionally. She gained weight and would not leave her house except to go to the doctors.

She came to see me for severe pain in her upper and lower back, hips and neck. She had been assured by the cancer specialists that there was no sign of active cancer in her body, either in the skeletal system or elsewhere. A back surgeon had told her that she had fairly severe spinal arthritis and disc disease that could be treated by surgery. She had already had many surgeries, some of which had permanent negative effects on bowel and bladder function. The spine surgeon could not guarantee that a surgery on her spine would successfully resolve her pain. She did not want another surgery. She was sure that if she did not have surgery her severe pain would continue for as long as she lived. This was quite depressing in itself. Pain management doctors had tried spinal pain blocks without success and could only offer her narcotics. But the narcotics only depressed her further without much relief of pain.

As part of my treatment, I had her see a clinical psychologist who has a great deal of experience with pain and the associated emotional states. My treatment focused on using manual medicine to rebalance a whole series of musculoskeletal imbalances that were contributing to her pain. I, too, spent a great deal of time listening to her litany of woes. I also started weaning her off the narcotics. Between my efforts and those of the clinical psychologist her mood began to improve. As her mood improved, so did her musculoskeletal pain. She suffered a brief setback emotionally when she finally had to move out of her house. At the same time, her musculoskeletal pain also got worse. Both were transient and she continued to improve. The last time I saw her she had only mild pain in her back and hips. Having dealt with her emotional issues her back pain occurred mostly when she got too aggressive about her new exercise program. She was even beginning to talk about going back to work.

PAIN AND POST-TRAUMATIC STRESS DISORDER

One of the hot-button topics in our society today is post-traumatic stress disorder (PTSD). This emotional problem probably has always been with us in one form or another but is much more visible as a result of the attempt of so many of our combat soldiers to return to civilian life. Essentially PTSD is an emotional response that is disproportionally large in response to a current event but is tied to previous events involving significant physical and/or emotional trauma. Most of the time that emotion is anxiety. In many, if not most cases, anxiety is tied to hyper-vigilance, hyper-reactivity and sometimes rage.

Although the case for emotional trauma as a cause for PTSD is fairly well accepted, it is the effect of physical trauma as a trigger for PTSD that is important to us in discussing somatic pain. Although the physical trauma triggering PTSD can be a single event, most of the time there are a series of physically and psychologically damaging events that lead to the development of PTSD. For instance, consider a soldier who has been involved in several firefights and/or explosions in which other soldiers in his platoon were severely injured or killed. Because of these events the soldier experiences strong anger and fear with every patrol. In the firefight that provokes his PTSD, his platoon is ambushed after an explosion overturns the vehicle in front of his. Shrapnel hits his back and left shoulder with some penetrating his left arm and shoulder. The rest did not penetrate his body armor, so no critical organs were damaged. Shortly after he recovers from his injuries his unit is rotated back from the area of conflict. He develops PTSD that is both physically and emotionally debilitating.

In PTSD the physical damage of the triggering event (or events) creates an additional component of strong negative emotion like anxiety, fear or anger. Each of these emotional states involves the release of adrenalin and noradrenalin into the bloodstream, as well as release of the same chemicals in the brain. In fact, there are recent studies that suggest that the use of medications that block the effects of adrenalin and noradrenalin in the body and brain (beta blockers) tend to prevent the development of PTSD.

One model that makes a great deal of sense is that the physical trauma and the negative emotional state get locked together in a form of learning. If we look at the case of my patient who tumbled down a mountain while skiing cited previously, one is struck by how much it resembles aspects of PTSD.

His original injury was quite damaging and potentially could have led to chronic pain and debility. It did not do so. However, later on in his life another trauma that resulted in much less physical injury provoked the development of intractable pain without any sign of a significant trigger. Because I was not thinking along those lines when he first came to me, it did not occur to me to ask if he was having any issues with fear, anxiety or anger at the time of his tumble down the mountain. Later on, he confirmed that his firm was going through particularly bad trouble around that time. He may have had a legitimate fear that his need for and response to narcotics would be seen as a reason to suspect his judgment and thus could further jeopardize his business. He had several reasons to have on-going fear and anxiety since there was the possibility that he could lose his business.

In the 1980's John Sarno, M.D., suggested that back pain was not only experienced in the person's head, it was, in fact, the result of abnormal emotional states. He originally based his hypothesis on the fact that treating those with chronic low back pain psychologically relieved most of their low back pain in 76 percent of the cases. Studies were beginning to suggest that disc herniation had no apparent relationship to the existence of low back pain. This seemingly confirmed Dr. Sarno's hypothesis. Subsequent studies have not confirmed such a high rate of treatment success using psychological tools alone. Nonetheless, Dr. Sarno's contention that back pain, and, by extension, most forms of musculoskeletal pain, are essentially psychosomatic (caused by the psyche) has entered popular literature and thinking.

In fact, as we have already seen, pain is not always present with injury. Further, acute and chronic pain is frequently associated with emotional states as noted above. In spite of Dr. Sarno's vigorous assertions, the concept that an emotional state is always the cause of chronic pain is not widely accepted in the medical and scientific communities. First, not all physical pain is associated with emotions. Many of my patients come to me with reports of musculoskeletal pain due to a minor injury like a fall or stepping off a curb inadvertently. They have pain. There is no fear, anger or even upset. They just want the pain to resolve. They know the cause of their pain. And they know that if they come to see me and get treated, their pain will go away.

Of course, there are those patients who have an emotional component to their body pain. Even in these people, the simple act of treating and correcting the physical (structural) triggers for pain is generally sufficient to stop both the pain and the resulting emotional response. That would not be possible if the mental-emotional disturbance was the actual cause of pain.

PAIN IS IN THE BRAIN

The complexity of the nervous system means that while the experience of pain looks simple, it is not simple at all. We get muscle reflexive responses to painful inputs that are quite unconscious and even difficult for us to prevent. We get sympathetic nervous system responses that are also unconscious. These add to the local pain receptor responses in the damaged tissue causing further dilation of blood vessels, reddening of skin or swelling and edema (fluid collection) in the damaged tissues. The sympathetic responses can also produce wider responses like increased heart rate, breathing rate, and blood pressure that will allow us to flee or fight if necessary to prevent further damage.

Because some of the complex pain pathways include outputs to emotional centers in the brain, the pain experience also can include significant emotional components. These emotional components then can color or change the meaning of pain. They may also make it harder for us to recover from an injury.

And finally, at many levels the signal can be stopped by feedback mechanisms, including some from the cerebral cortex itself. This is the reason that it may take a powerful input from the initial "injury" for us to experience pain or explain why the site of pain may change from one day to the next.

This same complexity in the nervous system also accounts for the fact that sometimes we can experience pain with very little, if any, present injury. As discussed earlier, sometimes pain occurs merely with the threat of injury. And, in some cases, there is no injury at all, although there may have been an injury in the past. Some of this exists because the nervous system is capable of learning or being predictive based on previous events. Some of the earliest experiments with animal learning involved the use of painful stimuli such as electrical shock paired with another stimulus that had no potential for injury. After repeated pairings of the painful and safe stimulus the animal will avoid the originally safe stimulus in order to avoid being shocked. This comes as no surprise. Human history is full of examples of pain being used to stop particular behaviors or to cause us to produce certain behaviors in order to avoid further pain. Unfortunately, in many cases the learned response also includes experiencing pain even when the painful stimulus is not present.

Aspects of this learning can even exist at the level of the spinal cord. One of the common findings in manipulative medicine is that reflexive restrictions in the spine and muscles are often easy to correct even when they have been present for a long time. However, particularly if the triggering event involved a fair amount of force or the restriction went uncorrected for a long time, it is easy for the restriction to return with only minor provocation. Part of the treatment method in manual medicine is to treat such restrictions repeatedly over time to help change the learned reflexes that have developed.

Finally, as suggested earlier, the complexity of the nervous system allows learned associations of all aspects of pain. Sometimes pain and depression or pain and anxiety can become so intertwined that the emotion immediately leads to the experience of pain even without an injury. Occasionally we see the development of abnormal associations of pain and pleasure. At another level we can see habitual avoidance of activities, thoughts, and even people and places that have become associated with pain. Because of its essential role in the functioning of the attention and emotion centers, the spinal cord and the thalamus and above all the cerebral cortex, pain can shape our very existence. Our pain and its meaning are literally in the brain.

CHAPTER 7
Managing Somatic Dysfunction and Inflammation

Living with muscle, tendon and/or joint dysfunction and pain is something most of us would rather not do. The prospect of living through part of a day in pain is bad enough. To wake up with pain and still have it our partner when we go to bed at night is distressing. Yet for many that is the shape of life.

One of the major points of this book is to allow those with chronic pain to find answers. There are several strategies that are used to decrease or eliminate pain. Some have been explored already. In this chapter we will look at strategies that are commonly used to manage or decrease pain and any problems connected to their use.

SURGERY AND PAIN

Surgery is one of the more common medical interventions for chronic pain. Frequently surgery is advised when there is muscle, tendon, joint, and bone restriction, clear evidence of major trauma, advanced arthritis and pain. The body part that needs surgical modification may have been altered by trauma or overuse. It may be torn or altered by arthritis. Surgery may change the structure enough to restore use of a bone or joint and diminish or abolish the pain. In the majority of cases this is sufficient.

However, surgery should never be entered into lightly. Torn tissue and bone can be sewed together and worn-out tissue can be replaced. However, surgery does not restore the body to a normal anatomical and physiological state. At the very least, scar tissue will form where there was none. Sewing tissue together will shorten it. Nerves may be damaged or even destroyed. Replacing bone with artificial material may produce something close to the original configuration, but because it is not living, it cannot adapt to change nor can it replace itself as it wears out. As the artificial parts wear out, they can further damage the surrounding tissues. Repeated surgery to replace artificial parts always results in further destruction of the surrounding tissues. Sometimes the artificial parts are significantly different from the natural parts they replace. And always, there is the possibility of infection. Thus, even the most skilled surgeon cannot completely restore tissue to its natural state.

There are two medical specialties dedicated to surgical correction of pain involving muscles, tendons, ligaments, joints, bone, and nerves. These are orthopedic surgeons and neurosurgery spine specialists.

ORTHOPEDIC SURGEONS

Orthopedic surgeons specialize in the surgical treatment of all muscle, tendon, ligament, bone and joint abnormalities, including those that produce pain. The general focus of orthopedic surgeons is on the bones and joints. Much of their work is dealing with problems stemming from injuries or the consequences of arthritis. The least invasive procedures typically practiced by orthopedic surgeons are injections. Other methods range from arthroscopic revision of damaged joints and tissues, surgically rebuilding shattered bones, modifying damaged spines, and joint replacement.

Arthroscopic surgery is part of the surgical revolution that took place at the end of the 20th century. Arthroscopic surgery is performed through small incisions through the skin. Very small video cameras are introduced into the structure so the surgeon can see what is happening. Other small instruments including probes, scalpels, drills, mills and suturing devices are introduced through additional small incisions to surgically treat the tissue without having to surgically open with a large incision. The two most common muscle and bone structures treated with arthroscopic surgery are the shoulder and the knee. In both cases arthroscopic surgery can be used to rejoin tendons that have been torn. It can also remove torn cartilage and even smooth or remove bone spurs and other irregularities on the joint that are causing restriction in movement and pain or fraying of the tendons. After healing from arthroscopic surgery and with sufficient physical therapy the joints are often usable with minimal pain or restriction for a long period of time. However, it should be understood that arthroscopic surgery does not replace structures that have been removed and over time the modified joint may go through arthritic deterioration.

When surgery is performed to correct bone fractures, it often involves placement of rods, plates and screws to help realign the bone fragments and allow an otherwise distorted structure with poor chances of healing the opportunity to return to normal or near-normal function. Typically, these surgeries involve larger incisions and can be quite complex. Sometimes the damage to a joint is extensive enough that the orthopedic surgeon must resort to older "open surgery" techniques with large incisions and more extensive surgical modification of the damaged tissue. The most common of these larger scale surgeries is the actual replacement of joints with artificial materials.

In addition to surgery for the limbs, some orthopedic surgeons specialize in surgery for the neck and spine. The most successful spine surgeries involve removal of herniated disc material and opening the nerve outlets. The most unsuccessful spine surgery is for lumbar spinal stenosis. While the initial success of spinal stenosis surgery is good at six weeks, the outcome at a year is typically not so good. Sometimes the surgeon's response is to do another surgery. Most often the second surgery has an even worse outcome than the first.

NEUROSURGICAL SPINE SPECIALISTS

The other group involved in spine surgery is the neurosurgeons who specialize in dealing with the problems of the spine and its enclosed spinal cord and nerves. Many of their procedures are similar to those of the orthopedic spine surgeons, although the focus of their training has been on the nervous system rather than muscles, tendons, bones, and joints.

OTHER MEDICAL SPECIALTIES THAT DEAL WITH PAIN

Other medical specialties that deal with the consequences of dysfunctions and pain of the muscles, tendons, bones and joints include interventional pain management (anesthesiology), interventional radiology, neurologists, physiatrists, psychiatrists, rheumatologists, and osteopathic neuromusculoskeletal specialists. Each of these specialists brings a different set of tools to the table. In many cases management of chronic pain will require doctors from several different specialties to get pain under control and help the patient achieve a better more functional level of existence.

Interventional Pain Management doctors are the only specialty that focuses exclusively on pain. They are trained in anesthesiology and most have taken subspecialty training in pain management. Typically, they use a number of different tools to help alleviate pain. These may include prescription of narcotics and other medications, nerve block injections, intra-spinal injections, nerve destruction (ablation), and implanted nerve stimulators.

Interventional Radiologists are radiology specialists who typically use needles inserted through the skin using x-ray and ultrasound machines to be able to see exactly where they are going. Like the interventional pain management doctors, they may perform joint injections, nerve block injections, injections inside the spine, and nerve destruction (ablation). If there is a spinal compression fracture that is no more than six months old, they may inject the fractured vertebra body with *cyanoacrylic* (superglue) to restore some of its height and stabilize it. The currently recommended version of this method involves injecting a balloon into the fractured vertebra body and inflating the balloon, which is filled *with* cyanoacrylic, a process termed *Kyphoplasty* that restores the vertebra to near normal and stabilizes it in a more appropriate shape. In doing so, they typically relieve the pain of the fracture almost instantly.

Neurologists are often an important part of the team effort in managing pain, particularly chronic pain. They often are called in as diagnosticians to determine whether the source of the pain is in the brain, spinal cord or in the peripheral nerves. They may use MRIs, CT scans, laboratory studies, and nerve conduction studies to tease out the root causes of pain. They also may perform nerve blocks and use Botox (botulinum toxin) injections to block muscle spasms.

Physiatrists or specialists in physical medicine and rehabilitation are kind of the jack-of-all-trades in the management of chronic pain. They are trained to manage physical therapy and rehabilitation programs. They often perform radiology guided injections, perform nerve conduction studies, and may prescribe narcotics as needed. Like the neuromusculoskeletal specialists, they often have a good working knowledge of the medical aspects of orthopedics and sports medicine.

Sports Medicine doctors can be from any of a number of specialties including orthopedic surgery, internal and family medicine, physical medicine and rehabilitation or neuromusculoskeletal medicine. They have additional training and have taken a qualifying exam focused on taking care of athletes. Although this is not a Board Certification in itself, it should indicate that the doctors focus at least part of their practices on musculoskeletal medicine and in some cases surgery.

Psychiatrists and Clinical Psychologists are often called upon to help people deal with physical pain. As noted above, pain and strong negative emotions are often intertwined. In some cases, it is difficult to change the neural and muscular, tendon and joint basis of pain without dealing with the psychological aspect of pain. Unfortunately, too often the medical profession will refer patients with chronic pain to psychiatrists because of the belief that the emotional states are causing the pain without adequately determining the cause or causes of pain.

Neuromusculoskeletal Medicine specialists like me are a very small minority in modern medicine. At this point in time, we are mostly osteopathic physicians although there is no intrinsic reason that M.D.s can't practice the same procedures, including treating with osteopathic manipulative methods. Most of us have additional postgraduate training in our specialty and many are, in fact, residency trained. In Europe there are a number of M.D.s who have decided to incorporate the osteopathic model and osteopathic manipulative treatment into their medical practices. They have taken postgraduate training in osteopathic medicine and manipulative treatment and are practicing as MD-DOs. Much of the idea behind what osteopathic physicians do and how we practice is contained in the first two chapters of this book.

Manual Medicine is the more general term for manipulative treatment applied to the muscles, tendons, ligaments, joints, bones, and neural tissue by physicians. Osteopathic manipulative medicine is the name given to the type of diagnosis and treatment utilized by osteopathic neuromusculoskeletal specialists. A number of M.D.s who have received musculoskeletal training similar to that of osteopathic physicians practice manual medicine outside of the United States. There are some in the United States as well. Some follow the diagnosis and treatment protocols developed by Dr. Janda in eastern Europe. Others base their manual medicine practice on models that have developed in their countries or regions, often from folk medicine sources.

OPIATES: AS BAD AS THEY ARE GOOD

One of the issues for many of the patients I have described has been the use of opiate narcotic medications to control pain. By opiate narcotics we are focusing on the morphine and codeine analogues and derivatives. There is no question that these medications do a good job of preventing the perception of pain, particularly acute pain. As we shall see, however, they are not without their problems.

Basically, all opiates work through the endorphin system of the body. As we previously discussed, endorphins are a class of neurochemicals that are released at the synapse by some neurons in the central nervous system. They also can be released into local tissues by the same neurons. Many of these neurons are found in the core systems of the thalamus, hypothalamus and brainstem where they are involved in controlling the pain pathways. They also are involved in the emotion and reward pathways of the hypothalamus and midbrain. Interestingly, they are also found in the local circuitry of the bowels where they are involved in the digestive processes. They are also found in the cells of the immune system.

When endorphins are released in the brain, they can do a good job of blocking the nerve pathways that bring pain information from the spinal cord to the thalamus and cortex. In fact, the release of endorphins is thought to be a significant part of the process involved in our normal methods for controlling pain. Endorphins also play a role in the development of pleasure, euphoria, and other rewarding emotions. This is undoubtedly the source of one of the big problems with opiates: addiction.

Opiates have been known for many centuries for their pain-relieving properties as well as for their pleasure and addiction properties. The milk of the opium poppy was used to relieve pain at least as far back as the Greeks and probably well before. In the Americas, the coca plant was used in a similar fashion long before the arrival of Europeans. By the later part of the 19th century, coca and opium derivatives were used in Western medicine for the relief of pain. Opium and alcohol concoctions were in wide use for minor pain relief and for relief of diarrhea. Even the original formula for Coca-Cola included derivatives from the coca plant. Both opiate and cocaine use were widespread, often having been started for the relief of pain but used persistently because of their addictive properties. By the 1930s the governments of the United States and many European countries had begun to crack down on the non-medical use of these drugs and their more potent derivatives like morphine, cocaine and heroin. Some were outlawed, while others were restricted to use under the prescription by medical doctors.

The properties of the opiates were well-known: pain relief, constipation, euphoria, and addiction. Opium and its derivatives tended to cause drowsiness and sleep, whereas cocaine could act as a stimulant. Otherwise, their effects were quite similar.

By the 1970s, the hypothesis was developed that the opiates were probably acting on the central nervous system through specific chemical receptors on the neurons. The discovery of the first of these receptor proteins in brain tissue by Solomon and Pert quickly led to identification of the natural chemical transmitters that would bind to these "opiate" receptors, the endorphins. Over the next 20 years, details were quickly discovered including the many specific pathways in the nervous system that used endorphins, locations of the sites of origin and release, determination of different versions of both the endorphin receptors and the endorphins themselves. The understanding of these complex pathways has resulted in a much better understanding of how the natural internal pathways work and why different opiates produce similar but varied effects.

The problems with using opiates to control pain revolve around several axes. These problems make it difficult to recommend any more than short-term use of opiate narcotics for the control of pain.

First, all opiates are to some degree addicting. Unfortunately, the problem of addiction itself is quite complex. There are several different senses in which the term "addiction" is used in relation to opiates. First, since pain is seen as something to avoid, the opiates can easily and quickly become a primary method of avoidance. This is a psychological dimension of addiction for those with pain. Second, the longer the opiates are used, the more likely that they will stop the natural production of endorphins. After between 20 and 30 days of more or less continuous use, the brain is no long producing endorphins. Thus, the normal pain control mechanisms used by the brain are stopped. The only way to control any pain, even that of a pinprick or a hangnail, is to use the opiates. Unless the opiates are used around the clock, pain will return whenever the level of opiates in the blood and brain drop below a certain level. Pain can then rear up and strike, even in the middle of the night, disturbing sleep. Third, because of the variations in blood levels, and the need to play "catch-up" in controlling pain, there tends to be an escalation of the dose needed to control the pain. One answer to these problems has been to develop long-acting opiate preparations, although necessarily these contain higher levels of opiate and thus are more subject to abuse. Finally, even though it is not as much of a problem in people who are in pain, the opiates are self-rewarding with their sense of euphoria and well-being. This emotional component is generally not viewed as being as much of a problem in pain management although it clearly is a big problem in the so-called recreational use of narcotics specifically for the associated high. Because of the addiction and abuse potential of the opiates all are classified as Scheduled drugs by the government of the United States. Their prescription by medical physicians is strictly controlled.

Used sparingly or briefly, most of the time opiates can be quite useful tools in dealing with pain. They work well to control acute pain when it threatens to overwhelm our natural internal pain control mechanisms. However, even with short-term use, opiates are not without potential problems. They almost always cause constipation. They also tend to cause a delay in gastric emptying so the whole gut is slowed down. If there is already a problem with gall bladder function, the opiates can make it worse.

Opiates also tend to slow reaction times and diminish mental sharpness, particularly during short-term use. Even though larger doses of opiates taken over a short time tend to produce euphoria, many find that chronic use tends to produce a sense of depression. Sometimes people in acute pain find these secondary symptoms sufficiently negative that they refuse to use prescribed opiates, resorting to non-opiate pain control methods instead.

More troubling in the use of opiates to control chronic pain is the fact that for some, chronic pain has evolved beyond what might be termed chronic re-injury. For these people, the opiates don't seem to do a good job of controlling their pain. Whether this is because the opiate receptors in the pain pathways have been essentially poisoned by prolonged exposure, or because pain has become a form of malignant memory rather than an actual activation of the pain pathways, is unclear. Whatever the cause, these patients do not seem to be helped by ever-increasing doses of opiates. Many of these patients do seem to have a heightened fear of pain at the same time, reinforcing their dependence on opiates for any relief they might bring.

As in short-term use of narcotics, an additional area of concern with the chronic use of opiates is the effect on the stomach and bowels. There are many endorphin nerves in the nervous system that control the activity of the gut. Most of them seem to slow the natural motion of the gut that propels food from one end to the other. For instance, it is well-known that taking must of the opiates tends to cause constipation. There is also considerable evidence that the narcotics can cause delayed stomach emptying (gastroparesis) and heartburn. They can also cause slowing of the normal emptying of the bile produced by the liver and concentrated in the gall bladder and might have similar effects on the pancreas.

Finally, there is a troubling aspect to opiate narcotics that I have seen in my practice that has not been researched at all as far I can tell. The longer the opiates are used to control pain, the slower the apparent healing of injured tissues. I suspect that part of the problem stems from opiate blockade at the level of the pain sensory neuron. Potentially such an effect could lead to problems similar to the destruction of pain sensors, namely diminishment of the natural healing response in the tissues. I am not even sure the effect is real. However, I can say that when my chronic pain patients go through surgery their tissue healing does seem to be less efficient and slow. Likewise, when I have a chronic pain patient who comes to my practice while on opiates, I can predict that they will take longer to resolve musculoskeletal restrictions than similar patients who are not on opiates.

Unfortunately, when patients come to me on long-term opiates to control their pain it is often difficult to convince them to go off their medicine. They all have had experiences where they have failed to take the opiate and their pain has gotten worse. Generally, it gets much worse. Even with many discussions about why this is true they are reluctant to face their pain. After all, in most cases stopping the opiate means pain will return with a vengeance, until their natural internal pain control mechanisms can get restarted. When this happens, after two to four days, most of the time the patient suddenly realizes that their pain is not that bad. In fact, in most cases there is hardly any pain. That is because their endorphins are ramped back up and pain can now be controlled by their normal internal mechanisms.

STEROIDS

Steroids are perhaps the most successful class of medicines used to manage pain outside of the opiates. They were developed based on a naturally occurring set of molecules in the body that are generated as the result of stress and trauma. Cortisone was the first purified steroid that seemed to block inflammation, whether from infection or injury. At the same time, it also seemed to dramatically decrease pain. The integration of pain and inflammation was discussed previously. Although pain can exist without obvious inflammation, virtually all inflammation includes pain. Because cortisone was so useful, it quickly became a priority to be able to synthesize it in the lab. There were several problems with this synthesized cortisone including the fact that it could only be delivered intravenously. Therefore, the race was on to develop other steroids that would have similar anti-inflammatory effects.

Fifty years later there are a number of anti-inflammatory steroids available. Prednisone and prednisolone are available in pill form as well as for injection. Most of the remainder of the available steroids are by injection only. Whether taken orally, injected locally, or injected into the circulatory system, all steroids are very effective at blocking inflammation throughout the body. They also seem to minimize pain that comes from inflammation.

Because many forms of arthritis are inflammatory in nature, steroids have long been a drug of choice in dealing with arthritis flares, particularly when the arthritis is of the auto-immune type like Lupus or Rheumatoid Arthritis. Steroids also help considerably with the inflammatory myositis syndromes, such as *polymyositis* and *polymyalgia rheumatica*. Injected steroids are also commonly used in joint and tendon injuries and bursitis. Their effectiveness in managing the occasional flares of osteoarthritis is generally not considered to be worth the risk so other medicines are used.

As good as steroids are at blocking pain and inflammation, they are not without problems. Taken for less than a month they may produce some general swelling, an increase in blood vessel fragility, and increased blood sugar, particularly in diabetics. Injected into joints and other circumscribed tissues they have the possibility of causing a weakening in the connective tissue after repeated use, so the general recommendation is to inject steroids into any particular joint of tissue no more than three or four times a year.

Taken for longer than 30 days, steroids may cause osteoporosis, increased fluid retention, weight and body fat gain, worsening control of blood sugar in diabetics, problems with the immune response and suppression of the body's own natural production of steroid. With prolonged use there is also an increased delay in healing and a decrease in our own natural response to stress.

In spite of these limitations, steroids are quite useful in managing pain and inflammation. When the situation is likely to be short-lived, steroids can produce rapid resolution of inflammation and pain. In other situations where the pain and inflammation are likely to be long-lasting, steroids can still be useful in lessening flares and, with careful management, can often be useful as an on-going treatment for pain and inflammation that cannot otherwise be controlled.

NON-STEROIDAL ANTI-INFLAMMATORIES

The non-steroidal anti-inflammatory medications, also known as NSAIDs, were developed as an alternative to steroids. Like steroids, these medications block both pain and inflammation.

The first non-steroidal anti-inflammatory medicine was actually developed in the 19th century. Aspirin, one of the most widely used medications in the world, was developed in German labs from the *salicylates* found in willow bark. Salicylate is a chemical that is not related to the steroids, but like the steroids has strong anti-inflammatory and pain-relieving properties. By chemically modifying the salicylate molecule, the chemists produced a powder that could be taken in a concentrated form orally. *Acetylsalicylic acid* is widely used for its pain-relieving properties, along with strong anti-inflammatory effects.

In the 20th century, new chemical compounds were developed that had anti-inflammatory and pain-relieving properties similar to aspirin but with some differences. Most are not chemically related to *salicylate* nor to the steroids but still have similar properties. These include *indomethacin, ibuprofen, naproxen, diclofenac* (Voltaren), *nabutenone* (Relafen) and *celecoxib* (Celebrex). Other NSAIDs have been developed over the years but have been removed from the human market due to their side effects, like *butazolidin*, and several of the Cox 2 inhibitors.

All NSAIDs block the formation of *prostaglandins*. Prostaglandin is a modified fatty acid that provokes very strong pain and is a major player in the development of inflammation. By blocking prostaglandin formation, both pain and inflammation can be relieved or even prevented. This makes the NSAIDs quite useful in managing both pain and inflammation.

NSAIDs have potentially significant side effects that frequently limit their use to a couple of weeks at a time. Major side effects include bleeding, bruising, gastritis, stomach ulcers, increasing blood pressure and kidney damage. In order to manage and prevent these side effects from developing it is generally recommended that the oral forms be taken no more than ten days in a row. Taking them on a continuous basis is much more likely to result in one or more side effects.

ACETAMINOPHEN

Acetaminophen (Tylenol, Paracetamol) is the only medication of its type available. Its precursor molecule, *phenacetin*, was widely used before the 1950s as an effective pain reliever. In fact, it was combined with aspirin and caffeine as the APC tablets used almost universally before the 1950s for headaches. When it was discovered that *phenacetin* was resulting in significant destruction of the liver, it was pulled from the market. A new and significantly less liver-toxic modification of the phenacetin molecule was developed and released in the late 1950s as Tylenol.

Acetaminophen is simply a pain reliever with a similar level of effectiveness to the NSAIDs. Acetaminophen does not work through the blockade of prostaglandin formation. Therefore, unlike the NSAIDs, it has no anti-inflammatory properties. Because of this, acetaminophen appears to be less effective when the issue is pain and inflammation but equally as effective as the NSAIDs at controlling simple pain. It is more effective than the NSAIDs at crossing into the brain through the so-called blood-brain barrier, so it has direct effects on the brain.

In the past few years, the possibility of toxicity developing with high doses of acetaminophen has become more public, although physicians have known of this possibility for years. Like its chemical cousin phenacetin, the primary negative effect of acetaminophen is on the liver. Phenacetin was a strong pain-blocking chemical that unfortunately turned out to be terribly toxic to the liver. As a result, it was removed from the market in the United States more than 70 years ago. Quite simply, at very high doses acetaminophen destroys the liver. For this reason, it is strongly recommended that adults limit their use of acetaminophen to less than 3000 mg per day. For children and small adults, the limit should be less. Also, drinking alcohol tends to magnify the liver destructive effect of acetaminophen, partly because the liver will modify the molecule back to phenacetin in the presence of alcohol. For these reasons, it is not advised to drink alcohol and take acetaminophen at the same time or even within five or six hours of each other.

COMBINED ACETAMINOPHEN AND NSAID

One of the surprising developments of the past few years is the practice of combining acetaminophen and an NSAID to help control pain. The aspirin-acetaminophen combination has been used for years for headaches, particularly when combined with caffeine. However, a number of studies have shown that combining naproxen or ibuprofen with acetaminophen can provide pain relief that is as potent as many of the opiates, even in post-operative pain. Since these medications are available over the counter and do not have any addiction potential, use of this combination is a good alternative both for acute and chronic pain. Of course, one must take care to avoid taking more than 2400 mg of ibuprofen or 1200 mg of naproxen and 3000 mg of acetaminophen in a 24-hour period. The NSAID and acetaminophen can be taken at the same time safely. Because of the gastritis potential of the NSAIDs they need to be taken on a full stomach.

BENZODIAZEPINES

The *benzodiazepines* are a class of medications that can be useful in pain management, although chronic use produces addiction. All work primarily in the brain. They can cause drowsiness, dizziness, muscle relaxation, poor coordination, memory loss and reduce anxiety. In some cases, they may cause mental changes. Because of their addiction potential and many potential side effects, these medications are used less for neural and muscle, tendon and joint pain syndromes than in the past. Librium (*chlordiazepoxide*), Valium (*diazepam*), Xanax (*alprazolam*), Ativan (*lorazepam*) and Klonopin (*clonazepam*) all tend to block anxiety and have muscle relaxing properties. Sometimes clonazepam is used in chronic pain syndromes when nothing else seems to help. Because of the abuse and addiction potential of these medications they are listed as Scheduled drugs by the government of the United States.

MUSCLE RELAXERS

The muscle relaxers as a class are useful in relieving muscle spasms that often accompany musculoskeletal pain. Typically, the more potent the muscle relaxation, the more likely they are to produce drowsiness and slowed reaction times. Presumably this occurs because much of their action occurs in the spinal cord and brain. Thus, the use of these agents is always a balancing act. The least effective and least likely to affect the central nervous system is Skelaxin (*metaxalone*). Stepping up in potency with still minimal sleep-producing effect is Parafon Forte (*chlorzoxazone*). There are four medications with moderate muscle relaxation effect and moderate drowsiness production: Zanaflex (*tizanadine*), Norflex (*orphenadrine*), Robaxan (*methacarbamol*), and Flexeril (*cyclobenzaprine*). Often these four are prescribed at a reduced dose during the day and at full dose at bedtime to promote sleep. Flexeril is chemically related to the tricyclic antidepressants (see sleep agents below). Soma (*carisoprodol*) is a little more potent than the other medications, but it also has a potential for addiction-type effects and has been listed in at least one state (Florida) as a drug with significant abuse potential. Lioresal (*baclofen*) is probably the most potent muscle relaxer and is known to have significant sleep-producing effects, so it is generally used with proven muscles spasms that are contributing to a significant pain-spasm-pain cycle.

NERVE STABILIZING AGENTS

There are two agents commonly used in pain management that have their origin in medications used to control seizures. Both are used to control the pain generated with nerve degeneration, termed neuropathic pain (see above). Neurontin (*gabapentin*) and Lyrica (*pregabalin*) both block specific calcium channels in the nerves, slowing their firing. They are particularly useful in peripheral neuropathies like those seen in diabetes and sometimes in idiopathic peripheral neuropathy. They can also be useful in helping manage chronic pain. Because this class of medications has shown some potential for abuse many states and even the Federal Government are now classifying them as Scheduled drugs like the benzodiazepines, opiates and sleep assisting medications

SLEEP PRODUCING AGENTS

The musculoskeletal injuries and imbalances that lead to pain often disrupt sleep. Poor sleep then prevents recovery from injury and in many cases makes the pain worse. One way to look at this complex circle is that sleep is a period of relative inactivity and relaxation that promotes healing. If pain keeps us from relaxing and letting the body and nervous system do what they need to do in order to heal properly, then our healing will be slowed.

There are two primary classes of medications used for sleep in such a case. The *benzodiazepine*-like medications: <u>Ambien</u> (*zolpidem*), <u>Lunesta</u> (*eszopiclone*), <u>Rozerem</u> (*ramelteon*), and <u>Sonata</u> (*zaleplon*) are generally prescribed for sleep disturbances. Ambien and Lunesta both are taken at the anticipated bedtime, last about eight hours and have some addiction potentials. Rozerem also lasts about eight hours but has little addiction potential and Sonata lasts about four hours and has minimal addiction potential. Each can be helpful in restoring a more normal sleep pattern in spite of pain. These medications are listed by the government of the United States as Scheduled drugs.

The other class of medications used for pain-related sleep disturbances are the tricyclic antidepressants, such as *amitriptyline* and *nortriptyline*, and a couple of other older antidepressants, *doxepin* and *trazodone*. All were classically used as antidepressants but had to be taken three times a day at doses that made the patient pretty groggy. Using them as sleep aids in pain syndromes once a day at bedtime takes advantage of their tendency to put the person to sleep. As a supplementary effect they will help with any pain-related depression. The tricyclic antidepressants can have side effects, particularly dry mouth. Also, all these medications tend to produce some persistent drowsiness after waking, particularly in the first week or two of taking them. Secondarily, all these agents tend to have stabilizing effects on peripheral pain nerves, so they also directly help with decreasing the pain signals particularly in neuropathic pain.

ANTIDEPRESSANTS

All modern antidepressants have been used to help with chronic pain syndromes. Some of the older antidepressants are now used primarily for their sleep-producing properties, but may have independent positive effects in controlling pain, particularly chronic pain. One of the positive effects of antidepressants is in relieving some of the negative emotions that stem from chronic pain and seem to make that pain worse. As discussed previously, one in particular, Cymbalta (*duloxetine*), has a specific indication for use in pain syndromes because molecularly it is close to Tramadol, a narcotic analogue, and has a mild pain-blocking effect along with its antidepressant effect.

CANNABIS

Cannabis, or marijuana, has long been known to have significant effects on decreasing pain as well as helping with glaucoma. Because of a long-standing policy of the United States government, it is classified as a Schedule I drug, or one that has significant abuse potential with no medical use. Because of this policy, little scientific research has been done on its pain-relieving properties. There is evidence that the cannabinoids have receptors in the central core of the brainstem that is known to transmit and modulate pain information. Hopefully the lack of scientific studies regarding the medicinal properties of marijuana and its derivatives will be rectified in the future. There has been a significant shift in public opinion on this matter and many states now allow medical use of this herb. On a state-by-state basis, marijuana is now being used to manage pain, musculoskeletal or otherwise.

There are two chemicals in cannabis that seem to affect pain. The more potent is *tetrahydrocannabinol* (THC). The second is *cannabidiol* (CBD). Medical marijuana contains both chemicals in specified concentrations. In those states that legally allow medical marijuana it is available by prescription from a licensed medical doctor.

Recently the U.S. Federal government allowed the growing and distribution of hemp. Hemp is related to cannabis, but by definition has less than 0.5% THC. Extracts from hemp contain varying concentrations of CBD. There is evidence that CBD by itself may be effective in controlling certain types of seizures, decreasing anxiety, helping with disturbed sleep patterns and helping control pain. It should be noted that, with the exception of certain seizure disorders, little controlled research has been published establishing the validity of claims for the effectiveness of CBD in other areas. However, anecdotal evidence does tend to support at least some of the claims being made about products containing CBD oil. The over-the-counter market currently offers oil extracts containing CBD. Unfortunately, because this market is unregulated, some of the products being offered may contain little or no CBD.

HERBAL MEDICINES AND NUTRACEUTICALS

In recent years it has become more and more popular to try alternative methods to improve general health and wellbeing. This includes the use of herbal medicines. There are a number of "natural" substances that have at least some effect on pain and inflammation. Some have been investigated in the laboratory. Others have at least anecdotal support for their effects.

White willow bark is the original source of *salicylic acid*, the progenitor of aspirin. Although white willow bark is not as potent as aspirin, it buffers the *salicylic acids* in a different manner than aspirin. Like aspirin, it has both anti-inflammatory and pain-relieving properties. Although it is less likely than aspirin to produce stomach irritation, it is probably not as potent a pain reliever.

Curcumin (Tumeric or cumin) is a very effective anti-inflammatory. It is probably more effective in the brain than most other anti-inflammatories, so it is receiving a lot of attention in treating brain inflammatory diseases such as Alzheimer's. The effective dose is 400 to 600 mg three times a day.

Green Tea has significant anti-oxidant and anti-inflammatory properties. There is evidence from laboratory studies that the *catechins* in green tea may also inhibit the breakdown of cartilage. This suggests that it may be useful in the treatment of osteoarthritis as well as in dealing with pain and inflammation. The usual recommended dose is 3 to 4 cups of green tea per day. As an extract, the dose is 300 to 400 mg per day. The decaffeination process does not appear to remove the beneficial *catechin* molecules.

Pycnogenol is extracted from Mediterranean Maritime Pine Bark. It has a strong anti-inflammatory effect but also tends to reduce clotting. Pycnogenol is extremely effective in the inflammatory aspects of heart and other circulatory diseases. It has a very strong anti-oxidant and anti-inflammatory effect. The usual dose is 100 to 200 mg per day.

Capsaicin is the active chemical that causes the burning sensation in chili and other hot peppers. Even though it stimulates the chemical burning sensation in pain nerves, it quickly depletes their ability to react to another painful stimulus. As a result, topical creams and transdermal gels that include capsaicin have proven quite useful in blocking those pain fibers that are fairly close to the skin.

Boswellia is also known as Frankincense. It has a strong anti-inflammatory effect as well as the ability to reduce auto-immune effects in the joints and other connective tissues. It has been used in the treatment of Rheumatoid Arthritis. Dosing is 300 to 500mg of standardized extract containing 30 to 40 percent boswellic acids per day.

Cat's Claw (*Uncaria Tomentosa*) is a Peruvian herb shown to block the primary inflammatory pathway. It should be used with caution by those with Lupus since it can worsen kidney function. Standard dose is 2060 mg per day or as a tea 1000 mg of root bark in eight ounces of water.

Ginger (*Zingiber officinale*) has long been used as part of the herbal pharmacy. It has been found in a couple of studies to relieve the type of muscle pain found with exercise. Although it probably does not have many direct anti-inflammatory or muscle-relaxing properties, it can significantly calm the stomach and smooth muscles found in the viscera. Since many of the anti-inflammatories, prescription, non-prescription and herbal, can cause stomach upset as a side effect, ginger can be particularly useful to help offset these side effects.

Devil's claw (*Harpagophytum procumbens*) is a South African herb that has long been used as part of folk medicine for the treatment of arthritis. It is thought to decrease the pain of arthritis and may even contribute to slowing the development of osteoarthritis although there are few scientific studies available in our medical literature to support such claims at this time.

St. John's Wort (*Hypericum perforatum*) is now widely known in this country for its use as an herbal anti-depressant. It has been shown in some studies to be as effective as many of the prescription antidepressants with significantly fewer side effects. Taken in conjunction with some of the other herbal treatments, it can be helpful in relieving some of the negative emotional effects of pain.

Valerian (*Valeriana officinalis*) is a plant from both Europe and Asia. It is commonly used to help relieve anxiety and promote sleep. There are few studies regarding its use for treating anxiety, but there is some data supporting its use as a sleep aid.

Kava Kava is a root herbal that is commonly used to relieve anxiety and help with sleep. In clinical trials it is modestly effective in both roles. However, it seems to have a significant liver toxicity resulting in it having been banned in some countries.

Omega 3 fish oil is produced by cold-distillation of the body oils obtained from fish, particularly cold-water fish. The undistilled fish oil also has Omega 6 and Omega 9 oils, and cholesterol. Cold-distillation removes all but the Omega 3 oils. A recent study published in the Journal of Neurosurgery demonstrated that Omega 3 fish oil at 3000 mg per day is as effective at blocking pain and inflammation as the maximum dose of ibuprofen (2400 mg per day).

The known side-effects of Omega 3 fish oil include:

1. Lowering LDL cholesterol (the so-called bad cholesterol)
2. Lowering triglycerides
3. Raising HDL cholesterol
4. Increasing vascular flexibility
5. Improving retinal function
6. Improving brain function
7. Blocking or slowing macular degeneration
8. Possibly slowing the progression of Alzheimer's disease
9. Decreasing the lung reactivity of asthma
10. Improving movement in the GI tract
11. Burping and increased gastroesophageal reflux.

All but the last are considered positive effects. In fact, cardiologists have recommended lower-dose Omega 3 fish oil (1000 mg per day) for a number of years because of its positive effects on cholesterol and the vascular system. The best way to avoid burping and reflux after taking Omega 3 fish oil is to take it at the beginning of a meal and avoid hot liquids until the end of the meal. An additional helpful trick is to put the fish oil in the freezer.

Omega 3 fish oil is available in 500, 1000, and 1200 mg capsules from many companies. Look for those that say either "tested for" or "certified free of" PCBs, mercury and heavy metals. The minimum anti-inflammatory dose is about 3000 mg of fish oil (1200 to 1500mg EFA+DHA). You can take up to 6000 mg per day, with increasing anti-inflammatory and pain-relieving properties with higher doses. It may reduce clotting a bit, particularly if you also take aspirin, Plavix or Coumadin/Warfarin.

Some have recommended taking Omega 6 fish oil along with Omega 3 fish oil. However, I do not recommend this for two reasons. First, Omega 6 fish oil *causes* inflammation. Second, there is too much Omega 6 oil already present in our diet (it is found in most vegetable oils). The problem is that there is not enough Omega 3 oil in our diet to balance all the Omega 6.

Although Flax Seed Oil also has an Omega 3 component that lowers cholesterol, it does not have any anti-inflammatory properties. I cannot recommend it for those who are trying to control pain and inflammation as well as generally improve health (see the listed side effects above). Recent data suggests that the Chia seed includes significant amounts of all three omega three oils. Therefore, it might prove to be a valuable vegetarian source of the anti-inflammatory omega 3 oils.

OTHER NON-MEDICAL PRACTITIONERS

There are several other types of practitioners who can be helpful in managing somatic pain and restriction. Some have extensive training and are licensed by the states in their limited practices. Others may have limited training or may not be licensed in their states.

CHIROPRACTIC

Chiropractic is a non-medical system of evaluation and treatment of muscle, tendon, and joint problems, particularly as they relate to the spine. It developed about the same time that osteopathic medicine did in the late 19th century in the American Midwest. Chiropractic rejected any connection with classical methods of Western medicine. Its basic premise was that many of the problems that drove people to see medical doctors had their origin in malfunctions in the bones, joints, muscles, and nerves, and most particularly dysfunctions and misalignments of the spine. The implication was that by correcting these imbalances or restrictions, the problems that would cause people to see medical doctors would also disappear.

In its more modern form, chiropractic focuses primarily on problems of muscle, tendon, joints, and bones. Chiropractic utilizes a series of methods to correct imbalances. The most common form of chiropractic treatment is based on thrusting maneuvers that cause some elements within the spine to make a cracking sound. By the latter third of the 20th century, a number of chiropractic practitioners have changed their methods of treatment to utilize less force, utilizing minimal force to achieve the rebalancing of muscle and skeletal elements. In some cases, their treatment methodology seems very similar to that of osteopathic medicine and physical therapy. Most patients that I have seen who had also seen chiropractors emphasize that the chiropractor focused their treatment largely on the area of pain.

In most cases, chiropractic physicians utilize X-ray studies and perhaps the results of MRIs to evaluate skeletal dysfunctions. Beyond radiological studies, chiropractic diagnostic tools differ significantly from those used in current medical practice. In many cases the conclusions drawn seem to be at variance with the diagnoses of current Western medicine.

Chiropractic training differs significantly from that of either the osteopathic or MD medical professions. They are licensed in each state by a chiropractic board. Although chiropractors generally tend to call themselves physicians, their training and practice is significantly different from the medical model. It includes different non-medical methods of diagnosis and treatment. Unlike MDs and DOs, Chiropractors are not licensed to prescribe medications or perform surgery.

That being said, many patients seem to benefit from chiropractic treatment. Particularly in the hands of more senior and experienced chiropractic physicians, results are sometimes quite good. Since there are many more chiropractic physicians than osteopathic physicians who practice musculoskeletal medicine, a limited course of chiropractic treatment for a particular episode of muscles and skeletal restriction or pain may be a reasonable alternative.

PHYSICAL THERAPY

Physical therapists are specialists in the rehabilitation of injuries to the muscles, tendons, ligaments, joints, bones, and nerves. All physical therapists have a bachelor's degree in physical therapy. Some have advanced degrees including master's and PhD's. They are licensed under a Board of physical therapy in all states. Their training and practice primarily focus on treatment and exercise rather than diagnosis. In general, they utilize more detailed analysis of physical restriction than that seen by medical physicians. The physical therapy emphasis is more on helping the patient achieve good functional status and minimizing pain and restriction. Some physical therapists have taken courses in osteopathic manipulative methods and use manipulative techniques that are virtually identical to those of osteopathic physicians who practice neuromusculoskeletal medicine. Along with some physiatrists and sports medicine specialists who use and prescribe exercise programs, physical therapy specialists are well-trained in using exercise as a treatment and maintenance methodology. A course in physical therapy managed by a physical therapist is often prescribed by medical physicians and surgeons after illness, injury, or surgery.

REHABILITATION AND SPORTS PRACTITIONERS, AND EXERCISE PHYSIOLOGY THERAPISTS

This is a diffuse group of practitioners most of whom operate under some form of license from the state. They are not physicians. Most have a very high level of practical training and experience. Frequently they are attached to professional sport teams where they provide the day-to-day management of inflammation and minor injuries. Their focus is on helping patients modify abnormal stance, walking and athletic activity that is either structurally unstable, causing pain, or is very inefficient.

In the past 30 years, a new profession has developed that formalizes this type of practitioner. Variously called rehab or sports physiologists, they have advanced degrees and formalized training. In Europe they are recognized as equal to physical therapists. At present there is no such formal recognition in the United States.

MASSAGE THERAPY

Massage therapy is a form of manual treatment focused on relieving tension in muscles and connective tissue. Massage therapists are licensed by the state in which they operate. Massage therapists must complete a course of study prescribed by the state in which they operate. Although many massage therapists may have college degrees, their license does not require it. Many have also taken advanced level courses. Massage therapists under law are not licensed as diagnosticians or physicians. They cannot prescribe a course of therapy. Sometimes they work with physical therapists. In most states they are allowed to operate independently. Some medical insurance policies will pay for massage therapy. Many others do not.

Massage therapy can be quite effective at relieving muscle and tendon tension. In doing so they may relieve pain. When the muscular and tendon pain is an effect rather than a cause, relieving the pain may be only temporary. As an adjunct to other forms of diagnosis and treatment, massage therapy can be quite useful in muscle and skeletal pain and restriction.

ACUPUNCTURE

Acupuncture is a method of diagnosis and treatment that utilizes very highly localized irritant forces to change the response of the body in disease processes. It has its origins in ancient Chinese medicine. The most common form of highly localized irritant used in Chinese medicine is the acupuncture needle. Other forms have been used including the use of suction cups (moxibustion) and electric current. The Chinese method is focused on correction of restrictions in what is termed Chi. Although Chi is not exactly synonymous with energy, life force, or the breath of life, it has elements of all three. There is no direct parallel in Western medicine to this form of diagnosis and treatment. There is mixed evidence that it is effective in its own right with some studies showing significant effect on managing pain and restriction. I have found it to be useful as part of a combined treatment regime for many patients.

There is a variant form of acupuncture that was developed in the United States that is termed medical acupuncture. This utilizes acupuncture needles inserted into identified tender points or trigger points as a treatment for muscle and skeletal restriction and pain. It is my experience that this form of treatment is less effective than traditional Chinese acupuncture or its variants from other Eastern countries like Japan or Southeast Asia.

EXERCISE AND STRETCHING TO MANAGE AND PREVENT PAIN

Throughout this book there is frequent reference to the use of exercise and stretching to both help manage pain and prevent pain and restriction. Many of the medical and nonmedical specialties that people turn to when faced with muscle, tendon, ligament, joint, and bone pain and restriction emphasize the use of exercise and stretching as part of their regimen for returning to normal function. From my standpoint, exercise and stretching, along with reasonable nutrition and good sleep, are the patient's essential contribution to their own restoration of health. Normally I will see a patient for half an hour more or less at a time and rarely more than an hour or two in a month. The remaining hours, days and weeks are in the hands of the patient. Although those of us who practice some form of manual treatment may restore balance to an out-of-balance musculoskeletal system, the only thing that is going to maintain that balance is a strong, flexible and healthy musculoskeletal system. To achieve that, the patient must exercise and stretch at least a few days a week.

CHAPTER 8
Arthritis

The most common cause for persistent pain in those of us over the age of 50 is arthritis. Pain in the joints is termed arthralgia. It is virtually certain that all of us will have suffered from arthralgia at some time in our lives. Arthralgia includes transient pain in a joint, pain in the joint due to injury, and pain from arthritis. It is important to remember that not all joint pain is arthritic. Furthermore, even though we frequently associate arthritis with joints, not all arthritis involves just the joints.

We assume that the pain from arthritis comes from inside the joint where one bone moves on another. Truthfully, most arthritis pain comes not from the joint surfaces but from the connective tissue around the joints, including the joint capsule, tendons and ligaments that cross the joint as well as the muscles that move the joints. Bone itself does not have many pain receptors. The connective tissue on the surface of bone, termed the *periosteum*, does have some pain receptors. So, too, does cartilage. However, most pain receptors found in the area of any joint are in the joint capsule and the tendons and ligaments that cross the joints.

JOINT STRUCTURE

Recall that the purpose of a joint is to allow two neighboring bones to move relative to each other. As was first discussed in Chapter 2 the joint is a complex structure. The bone faces are frequently rounded heads or receiving sockets at the end of the bones. The bone faces are covered by cartilage, a smooth, dense and somewhat flexible form of connective tissue. Between the two cartilage-covered bone faces is joint fluid that provides a slick interface between the two surfaces (see fig. 2-3).

A joint capsule made up of tough connective tissue encloses the ends of the two bones (see fig. 2-2). It is flexible enough for the joint to move but strong enough to keep the bones from separating. It keeps the joint closely packed and keeps the fluid within the joint. The joint capsule also includes tissue that generates joint fluid and absorbs it when needed.

JOINT FLUID

The specialized cells that create the joint fluid line the inner surface of at least part of the joint capsule. Joint fluid is not like blood. It normally has no red blood cells or white blood cells. It is also thicker than blood because it contains specialized proteins that help make it slick, keeping the surface of the cartilage slick and lubricated, similar to the role of oil between moving metal parts.

When too much joint fluid is produced it swells the joint capsule, generating pain. If it swells too much, a partial rupture of the bag can occur, like a swelling bubble on a tire. A Baker's Cyst on the back of the knee is one such example. Similar to that are the ganglion cysts sometimes seen around the wrist.

LIGAMENTS

Ligaments are well-organized fibrous bands that cross the joint from one bone to the other. Ligaments always act to limit how much the joint can move. Sometimes the ligaments are outside the joint, like those on the inside and outside surfaces of the knee, the medial collateral ligament and the lateral collateral ligament. They keep the two bones of the knee joint from moving too far medial or lateral relative to each other.

Inside some joints there are also tough ligaments between the bones that keep the bones from slipping too much. The anterior and posterior cruciate ligaments in the knee are examples. These ligaments keep the upper bone of the knee joint (femur) from sliding too far forward or backward on the lower bone, or tibia.

TENDONS AND MUSCLES

Muscles and their tendons cross most skeletal joints. The muscle causes the bones to move relative to each other. Recall that muscle consists of fibrous tissue that surrounds the active movement-generating elements, the muscle cells. At the ends of each muscle the fibrous tissue thickens into tendons that attach to bones on either side of the joint. In a few cases, a muscle may cross more than one joint in order to provide movement of more than one joint.

As noted earlier, the connective tissue surrounding the muscle cells, and more particularly the tendons, contains many nociceptors. So too do the joint capsules and ligaments. In each case the primary function of the pain receptors seems to be as a warning system when too much stress is being put on the joint or as an indication of joint failure.

BURSA

Bursa is the Latin word for sack. Bursae (plural) are found around most joints. They are out-pockets from the joint with a fibrous outside and an inner lining identical to that seen in joint capsules. They are typically seen lying under tendons in a pattern to keep the tendon from rubbing on other tendons or the underlying bone. Normally the pockets are flat with a very minimal amount of joint fluid between the upper and lower inner surfaces. This allows the bursa to act like a glide bearing so the tendon can move smoothly over other tendons or bone without rubbing or getting frayed.

Occasionally the inner pocket of a bursa develops inflammation. There is increased fluid causing swelling in the bursa and because the fluid is inflammatory the bursa becomes painful. Bursa inflammation is termed bursitis. Contributing to the pain of bursitis is what appears to be a contact inflammation in the overlying tendon(s) and the underlying bone surface. In many cases bursitis develops seemingly spontaneously and is termed idiopathic. In other cases, there has been a blow to the overlying tissues and bleeding develops in the bursa. Blood cells then cause the bursa to produce additional inflammatory fluid producing traumatic bursitis. One of the most common sites of bursitis is over the lateral aspect of the hip (the greater trochanter of the femur). Other common sites include the knee and the elbow. Treatments vary, but as a rule oral and topical anti-inflammatories are minimally effective. The most effective treatment is injection with steroid into the bursa.

ARTHRITIS AND THE JOINT

The most common form of long-term damage to the joint and the tissues surrounding the joint is arthritis. Often arthritis causes pain. Since the cartilage of the joint has very few pain receptors, most of the pain comes from the tissues around the joint. Pain can occur because these tissues are inflamed or because they are having to work overtime around a joint in a difficult rather than smooth motion.

The damage that arthritis produces can take several forms. The most common form of damage is the wearing down and fraying of the cartilage surfaces between the bones. This is termed osteoarthritis. The second is an actual erosion of the bone within the joint capsule. This kind of arthritis occurs as the result of the immune system attacking the joint tissues. It is known as autoimmune arthritis. The third type of arthritis comes from the development of calcium or other mineral deposits in the joint capsules, tendons and ligaments. This is termed crystal arthritis.

OSTEOARTHRITIS

Osteoarthritis is the most common type of arthritis. Its hallmark is the erosion or wearing down of the cartilage that forms the smooth surfaces between the bones. When cartilage on the bone surfaces is thick and smooth it allows easy movement between the bones. As a rule, cartilage does not repair itself nor does it regrow. As this cartilage wears down it gets thinner. More important, the cartilage surfaces become frayed. When the cartilage surface is rough, it catches on the other roughened surface. This sandpaper action accelerates the breakdown of the cartilage every time the joint is moved. When cartilage frays or breaks down, it is a one-way process.

As the cartilage thins and roughens, movement across the joint becomes more difficult. The muscles must work harder to achieve the same motion. Eventually the cartilage can wear out completely. This is the classical "bone-on-bone" situation that frequently leads to either a joint with very limited range of motion or the need for surgical replacement.

Osteoarthritis can occur in virtually any joint of the body. It is more common in those joints that are subject to chronic or reoccurring stress like the knees, hips, feet, spine, shoulders, and fingers, especially the thumbs. In the hands it initially presents most often as pain and stiffness in the thumb as it joins the bones of the wrist and the finger joints. As it progresses, the finger and thumb joints can swell and become deformed. Eventually they may even fuse. Enlargement is also common in the joints of the feet and knees. In the hips and shoulders, the primary symptoms are limitations of normal motion and pain with use.

The pain that accompanies osteoarthritis is often assumed to be due to inflammation in the joint. It is true that inflammation does occur at times in the osteoarthritic joint, particularly after overuse. Naturally, when inflammation occurs it will produce pain. However, contrary to popular belief, the osteoarthritic joint is not inflamed most of the time. Therefore, most of the pain in these joints is not the result of inflammation. It is common to use oral anti-inflammatory medications like ibuprofen or aspirin to help with the pain of osteoarthritis. Although it does help with the pain, it is not because it is blocking inflammation.

Actual pain from the abrasion of cartilage in the joint is rare because there are relatively few pain receptors in the cartilage. Rather, as suggested earlier, most of the pain in osteoarthritis comes from two other sources. First, the erosion of cartilage sometimes produces an increase in the fluid within the joint. This acts to buffer the joint surfaces by separating them further. However, the increased swelling within the joint puts a lot of pressure on the joint capsule and sometimes on the tendons and ligaments around the joint. This stretches these tissues for a long time. The joint capsule, tendons and ligaments have many pain receptors. Persistent stretching of these tissues is one of the activators of pain.

The other factor in causing pain in the osteoarthritic joint is the stiffening of the joint due to the roughening of the surface of the cartilage. Because the joint is harder to move, the muscles around the joint must work harder and exert more strength to produce the same motion that was easy to do when the joint was normal. This puts more stress on the muscles and tendons. That stress will produce pain from the muscles and tendons that cross the joint.

The deposition of calcium or other minerals in the soft tissues of the joint is also a characteristic of osteoarthritis. It is not clear why calcium deposits form around joints. One possibility is that they are the result of transient episodes of inflammation as the body deals with an increasingly arthritic joint. Whatever the cause, after many years of over-stress of joints it is quite common to see heavy deposits of calcium develop, particularly where the soft tissue connects to the bone. Sometimes these deposits can be so heavy that the actual joint appears enlarged and deformed. On an X-ray, the soft tissue calcifications are often seen as "spurs." Even though such spurs are often viewed as being related to the bone itself, anatomically it appears that most are actually calcifications of the soft tissue where it inserts onto the bone. This can be true at the joint capsule, the tendons and ligaments. The spurs themselves rarely produce pain. However, when the surrounding tissues are pressed into a spur, pain will often be felt. The classic example is the bone spur on the heel of the foot. The calcification is on the system of tendons and ligaments that form the plantar fascia binding bones together to form the sole of the foot. After prolonged stress to the plantar fascia, calcifications form in the fascia where they attach to the heel. On an X-ray it looks like a spur. Standing on the foot puts pressure on the skin and other connective tissue that covers the heel and fascia. The pressure of the overlying skin and connective tissue on the spur produces pain. The exact source of the pain in this case is unknown. Some may be from the tendon or ligament itself since its junction with the bone is no longer flexible. Possibly some of the pain comes from the overlying tissues rather than from the spur itself.

Often it is assumed that osteoarthritis stems from overuse of the joint. This would suggest that we should use the osteoarthritic joint less. In fact, that is what many of my patients have assumed over the years. However, not using an arthritic joint will result in weakening of the muscles and tendons around the joint. Disuse atrophy will then cause more pain because when we try to use it the weakened tissues are no longer up to the job of moving the joint. We often see this in older people whose arthritis is approaching the bone-on-bone stage. There is visible atrophy of the muscles and the joint is immobilized. Others, who have continued to use the severely osteoarthritic joint show no muscle and tendon atrophy and may not even have pain.

Some years ago, a 60-year-old woman came to my office suffering from low back and hip pain that started with a motor vehicle accident about four months before. Her story speaks to the issue of osteoarthritis and atrophy of the surrounding muscles and tendons. This patient had been physically active prior to the motor vehicle accident. She was involved in intense daily aerobic exercise and sports. She had never had any back or hip pain. Immediately after the accident she had some low back pain. As a result, she was taken to the Emergency Room for evaluation. They could find little wrong with her back and concluded that she had suffered only minor soft tissue damage to her lower back. However, the X-rays showed that both of her hip joints were bone-on-bone. My patient was very shocked by this finding since her hips had never given her any problem. The ER doctor advised her to go home and rest. He also insisted that she should not continue her daily exercise routine. He instructed her to follow up with an orthopedic surgeon within a few days.

The orthopedic surgeon told her that her hips had end-stage osteoarthritis and needed to be replaced. Now remember that she had never had any hip pain prior to the accident. In fact, she still was not suffering from any hip pain. Nonetheless, the surgeon told her she should schedule surgery with him within the next month or two. He did tell her about all the possible complications of the surgery and the problems associated with the hip replacements over the long term. He instructed her to go home and rest. Again, she was specifically instructed not to exercise her hips. While she was not happy with the prospect of surgery, she did listen to the doctor's instruction. She felt that if she resumed exercising it would make her arthritis worse.

Over the next several months my patient continued to have some discomfort in her low back. Worse, for the first time she developed pain in her hips. That is when she came to see me. Her back pain was easy to treat and resolve. Unfortunately, after four months of disuse she was developing significant atrophy and weakness around her hips. Attempts to return her to her prior exercise routine were thwarted by severely increased pain any time she tried. Finally, she gave in and had the surgery. Last I heard from her she was back to her old exercise routines and doing well.

As suggested previously, the common belief even among doctors, is that osteoarthritis is the result of overuse of a joint. The problem is that joint cartilage does not have good blood supply and is very slow to repair itself if there is any damage. Also, the repair process seems to get worse as we age. Other factors that appear to affect the ability of cartilage to repair itself are congenital abnormalities in the proteins that make up cartilage, metabolic diseases like thyroid disease and diabetes, and malnutrition.

Prolonged compression of a joint seems to accelerate cartilage degeneration. Thus, being significantly overweight can produce cartilage degeneration in weight-bearing joints like the knees and hips. While some of the overweight people I see have early osteoarthritis in these joints, the proportion of those over 65 who had to have knee replacements is much higher than those who are not overweight.

Injuries to joints can also accelerate the type of processes that lead to osteoarthritis. Consider what happened to another of my patients. At age 42 he suffered an injury to his left knee in a skiing fall. It was diagnosed as a complete tear to the medial meniscus of his knee. There are two cartilages in the knee that are separate from the cartilage that covers the bone surfaces of the joint. Each of these two cartilages is shaped like a new moon and is termed a meniscus. There is one on the outside and one on the inside of the knee joint. They help turn the lower flat surface of the tibia into more of a receiving cup. When they tear, they become a major irritant within the knee. With a complete tear the orthopedic surgeon had to remove his medial meniscus surgically. When I saw this patient years later his right knee was normal but his left knee was severely arthritic, particularly on the middle side of the joint. Presumably both the initial injury and the abnormality caused by the surgery had accelerated the breakdown of the surface cartilage of his joint.

The one form of osteoarthritis that is clearly related in joint injury is traumatic arthritis. Even without surgery when a joint has been injured, we are more likely to see rapid development of what looks and acts like osteoarthritis.

Consider the case of another of my patients. At 41 she retired from 20 years as a military pilot. At her last preflight physical just a couple of months before retirement, she had routine X-rays of her spine. They were entirely normal. A month after she retired, she was a passenger in an automobile accident. She broke no bones but suffered lot of bruising and developed pain in her neck, low back and right hip. The Emergency Room took X-rays again to be sure she had suffered no fractures. These, too, were normal. Seven months later when the pain in her neck persisted in spite of physical therapy, she came to see me. Her neck and low back seemed unusually stiff and, in spite of my best efforts and her willingness to exercise, the pain persisted. After a month I felt that perhaps we had missed something in the original studies from the Emergency Room. Therefore, I ordered an MRI of her neck and low back. I also requested the radiologist to compare the MRI to the previous X-rays. Much to my surprise the radiologist reported that she now had significant disc degeneration and arthritis in both her neck and low back, findings which had not been present eight months prior. She had developed traumatic arthritis.

We see the development or early major arthritis in the knees and hips of many professional athletes ranging from football players to gymnasts.

Their arthritis may require joint replacement in their 30s and 40s rather than their 70s. Presumably the acceleration of joint damage is from significant traumas suffered while competing in sports. Traumatic arthritis looks and acts like osteoarthritis but develops over a relatively short period of time. Osteoarthritis, it seems, may involve the accumulation of many small traumas over time rather than all at once.

AUTOIMMUNE ARTHRITIS

In some situations, immune responses of the body seem to attack parts of the bone inside the joint or even components of the joint capsule and surrounding tissues. This is the class of diseases termed autoimmune arthritis. These immune attacks on the joints and surrounding tissues do involve active inflammation which produces pain. If the immune attack on the joints and/or surrounding tissues goes on for a long time it typically leads to the joint becoming deformed. The deformity and resulting decreased range of motion also produces a strong component of pain. Autoimmune arthritis takes a number of forms including rheumatoid arthritis, lupus arthritis, Sjögren's syndrome, Polymyalgia rheumatica, Crohn's-related arthritis, psoriatic arthritis, and Myositis syndrome. Sometimes people who suffer one form of autoimmune arthritis also have Hashimoto's thyroiditis (see next chapter).

Autoimmune arthritis in all its forms may have a significant genetic component. However, the link is not so tight that if a relative had one of these diseases you will inevitably also have it. It appears that stress and other environmental factors also play a role in developing these diseases. For instance, I had an acquaintance years ago whose great aunt had rheumatoid arthritis, even though no other relative had the disease. My friend was in her early 40s and had always enjoyed good health. When both her mother and grandmother died within months of each other and then the IRS audited her, she developed diabetes, hypothyroidism, and rheumatoid arthritis by the end of that year.

RHEUMATOID ARTHRITIS

The most common autoimmune arthritis is rheumatoid arthritis. The initial attack of rheumatoid arthritis is most commonly on the knuckle joints of the hands (*metacarpophalangeal* joints). Most of the time, the following attacks are marked by pain, swelling, tenderness and reddening of the overlying skin on one or more of these joints, often the same joint on both hands.

In most cases, laboratory tests for inflammation (sed rate or C-reactive protein [CRP]) will be elevated during a rheumatic flare) will show the presence of rheumatoid arthritis. In most cases, laboratory tests for rheumatoid factor (RF) will be elevated whether there is an active flare or not. The hallmark X-ray sign of rheumatoid arthritis in the joints is erosion of the bone inside the joint leading to a decrease in the actual amount of bone-to-bone surface.

The disease can attack any joints but is most commonly seen in the hands and feet. It rarely visibly attacks the joints of the fingers themselves but can lead to the fingers being angled away from the thumb. Rheumatoid arthritis is a chronic disease. That is, once it develops it rarely goes away. However, it can vary in how active it is over time. At times it can be quiet with little active inflammation. At other times it can show quite active inflammation, often called a flare.

It used to be said that from the time rheumatoid arthritis developed the person had a life span of about 10 years if untreated. This was probably an exaggeration although the untreated disease can eventually spread to other organs, particularly the heart and blood vessels. Over the last 20 years the treatments for rheumatoid arthritis have advanced a lot. It used to be that treatment was initiated with anti-inflammatory medications, whether steroids or NSAIDs. Another medication, termed a DMARD (disease modifying anti-rheumatic drug) would be added after the disease had progressed to the point where the person had pain even with anti-inflammatory medications. Today the standard of care is to initiate treatment with both an anti-inflammatory and a DMARD.

Recently the class of DMARDs has been expanded to include biologic agents that block the pathways leading to tissue inflammation and erosion. These newer DMARDs are frequently aimed at blocking tumor necrosis factor (TNF), a naturally occurring substance in the body used to destroy cancer cells and invading organisms. TNF is significantly higher than normal in many types of autoimmune arthritis including rheumatoid arthritis. Blocking TNF seems to be quite effective in blocking the progression of rheumatoid arthritis. Most of the medications in this class do have several side effects, the most worrisome being suppression of the normal immune response to invading organisms.

The intent behind using DMARDs early in the development of rheumatoid arthritis is to slow or stop the progression of the disease. The success of this strategy is measured by both pain relief, diminished or absent flares, and lack of progression of joint erosion. It has made rheumatoid arthritis much less fearsome and much less painful.

Juvenile rheumatoid arthritis (JRA) is a variant of rheumatoid arthritis. It is found in children typically between 6 and 16 years old and often occurs after a bacterial or viral infection. It is more likely to affect large joints like knees and elbows as well as hands and feet. It may involve a single joint or many. The joint(s) become red, painful and swollen. Its treatment is similar to that for normal rheumatoid arthritis.

LUPUS, SJOGREN'S, CROHN'S AND PSORIATIC ARTHRITIS

Other forms of autoimmune arthritis diseases also include inflammation in other tissues as well as joints. The arthritic component of each looks similar to that in rheumatoid arthritis. That is, the joints can be severely inflamed and become eroded over time.

In Systemic Lupus Erythematosis (generally termed Lupus) the same attack can occur in a number of the non-musculoskeletal organs, particularly the kidneys, skin, heart, lungs and blood cell-forming system. Frequently the presenting signs are painful joints coupled with a rash on the face involving both cheeks and the bridge of the nose. This "butterfly rash" is considered a leading sign. However, it can be confused with other facial rashes and is not always present. Lupus is primarily diagnosed by a series of antibodies that collectively are termed the lupus antibodies. If it is not treated, Lupus can be a very debilitating and sometimes fatal disease, mostly due to damage of the internal organs. As with rheumatoid arthritis, the DMARDs are a key to the successful management of Lupus.

In Sjögren's disease there is significant arthralgia or joint pain. It may not show as strong an inflammatory flare as rheumatoid arthritis, but over the long run it can produce significant joint damage. Its other sign is a dry mouth and dry eyes. The damage seems to be to the fluid-producing cells in the tear ducts and saliva glands. It can also produce lung inflammation, lymph-node enlargement, and kidney, nerve, and muscle degeneration. The classic blood markers are the Sjögren's antibodies. Again, treatment involves use of DMARDs.

Crohn's disease involves the development of inflammation in the small and large intestines. Not everyone who has Crohn's disease develops arthritis. However, when they do the arthritis is inflammatory and erosive similar to that in cases of rheumatoid arthritis.

Similarly, psoriasis is primarily a disease of the skin. Psoriasis does not always involve the development of arthritis. As with Crohn's disease, an inflammatory arthritis may also develop.

POLYMYALGIA RHEUMATICA AND MYOSITIS SYNDROME

When the inflammation around the joints involves the muscles and tendons rather than the joints themselves, the result will be pain that is not localized to the joints. Instead, it seems to be all over.

In Myositis Syndrome, the inflammation seems to be in the muscles themselves. It is not clear whether it is in the muscle cells or in the connective tissue that surrounds muscle cells and gives them their leverage to shorten and move the joints. There are particular blood markers that suggest Myositis. The degree of inflammation and its severity varies from person to person. In extreme cases the attachments to the tendons can weaken and even tear. In some cases, severe calcium deposits can form in the muscles and tendons.

Polymyalgia Rheumatica is a different inflammatory disease than Myositis Syndrome. The only characteristic is widespread muscle pain and elevation of the blood markers for inflammation (Sed rate or C-reactive protein). Over time there can be a significant weakening or even atrophy of muscles. There is no evidence that this is caused by nerve degeneration. Rather it is a problem in the muscles themselves. The only treatment so far is to use steroids. Steroids can stop and reverse the progression of Polymyalgia Rheumatica. Control of the disease may or may not require chronic use of steroids.

CRYSTAL ARTHRITIS

The most common form of arthritic mineral deposit that can form in the connective tissues around a joint is uric acid. When the level of uric acid in the blood is too high for too long it will sometimes develop into large uric acid crystals in the connective tissues around the joint. When the load of uric acid crystals is too great, they can form a large inflamed lump in the tissue termed a gouty tophus (*pleural tophi*). In joints with *gouty tophi* there are also increases in uric acid within the fluid of the joint. As that occurs the joint becomes red, hot to the touch, swollen and very painful. This is termed a gout attack. Gout affects the big toe most frequently but it can affect other toes, the ankle and hands. It will rarely attack the large joints like the knees.

The primary way to abort a gout attack is to put the patient on a strong anti-inflammatory medication like *Indomethacin* or a steroid and as well to use *colchicine*, a medication that seems to help speed the recovery from a gout attack. A person with gout is often urged to avoid red wine and organ meats since they tend to increase uric acid. The primary way we can prevent gout is to bring the blood levels of uric acid down to normal and keep it there. The primary medicine used to lower uric acid is *Allopurinal.*

One form of calcification seen commonly in connective tissue around a joint is very small deposits, like sand, scattered within the tissue. When these types of calcium deposits are particularly dense in the tissues around the joint, an arthritis flare can occur in that joint. When it does, there is very significant pain, swelling and redness in the skin over that joint. It looks almost exactly like gout. However, the person who is suffering from this joint inflammation does not have a high uric acid level in the blood and no uric acid crystals in the joint. This form of arthritis is termed pseudogout. The most common treatment is to use an anti-inflammatory medicine like an NSAID or steroid.

Although it is not clear what mechanism drives the deposition of these particles, it does seem to relate to persistent stress on the affected joint. Perhaps it is similar to the kind of mechanism that causes the development of the *sesamoid* bodies within tendons where they cross some joints. These sesamoid bodies typically develop after birth and are generally fairly small. The most common are seen in the tendons in the palm of the hand and soles of the feet, although the largest is the knee cap. Sesamoid bodies are not arthritis but rather an organized calcium deposit within a tendon as it crosses a joint.

CHAPTER 9
Muscle Pain and Myalgia

Myalgia is literally pain in muscles. Actually, much of the pain in our muscles comes from the connective tissue that surrounds and is embedded in the muscles and the ligaments that attach the muscles to bone.

Remember, the actual muscle cells do not have pain receptors. However, the connective tissue carries blood vessels and nerves that supply, control and sense what is going on with the muscle cells. These pain sensory neurons are embedded in the connective tissue.

There are a number of reasons why these pain sensory neurons can be activated. When the muscle cells are active too long their supply of oxygen and blood sugar may no longer be sufficient. They produce too much lactic acid which leaks from the muscle cells into the surrounding tissues and local veins. Other metabolic waste products are also released into the surrounding tissues. Extra muscle activity may overwhelm the ability of the blood flowing away from the muscles to carry off all the wastes produced. The increased lactic acid and other metabolic waste products produce inflammation and cause the nociceptors to fire. However, the pain resulting from muscle overuse in sports is rarely strong. It would not be classified as myalgia.

Myalgic pain is both relatively strong and persistent. It can be strong enough to keep us from further physical activity. Unfortunately, in many cases it is active even when we are not. It can range from being merely irritating to searing and burning. There are a number of potential causes for myalgia. Some people develop it because of endocrine disorders and others because of medications. A third group develops myalgia as a part of an arthritic condition, particularly of the autoimmune variety. Finally, there is a fairly substantial group who suffer from fibromyalgia. It is important to determine that a person does not have one of the first three causes for their myalgia before giving them the diagnosis of fibromyalgia. Treatment for each potential cause of myalgia is different, as is the possibility for successful resolution.

ENDOCRINE DISORDERS AND MYALGIA

The most common endocrine cause for myalgia is thyroid disease. The thyroid gland is considered the master of metabolism. Thyroid hormones are necessary for the use of blood sugar and fats in most tissues. The thyroid can be underactive (hypothyroid) or overactive (hyperthyroid). Both states can produce muscle pain. Both can be readily diagnosed by blood tests that evaluate thyroid stimulating hormone (TSH) levels and the levels of T3 and/or T4, the active thyroid hormones.

If TSH is low and either T3 or T4 are high, the person is diagnosed as hyperthyroid. Typically, there will be an increase in appetite with accompanying weight loss. Anxiety is frequently present. The heart tends to race and blood pressure may be elevated. And, of course, myalgia is present, in part because muscles tend to be tensed all the time. Treatment is most commonly the destruction of the thyroid gland or use of suppressing medications. The myalgia and other symptoms of hyperthyroidism will generally disappear with successful treatment.

If TSH is high and T3 and/or T4 are low the person is hypothyroid. Gaining weight is common and losing weight seems to be impossible. They might feel fatigued with no energy or even somewhat depressed even though there is no real reason to be depressed. Like those with the hyperthyroid condition, people who are hypothyroid can have myalgia, although for a different reason. The lack of the thyroid hormone lowers the metabolism and ability of muscles to use blood glucose to produce the energy needed to function. Since we have to use our muscles in any case, metabolic failure leads to muscle pain. The treatment of hypothyroidism involves use of a prescribed thyroid hormone. Although the process of achieving proper levels of thyroid hormone can take time, once the blood levels are essentially normal, the symptoms of hypothyroidism resolve, including myalgia.

The third thyroid problem that can lead to myalgia is a genetic disease called Hashimoto's Thyroiditis. In my practice, Hashimoto's has been one of the most frequent causes of myalgia that has been missed or mislabeled by other doctors. For years Hashimoto's was thought to be one of the rarest thyroid diseases. If it was diagnosed at all it was because the surgeon removed part of all of the thyroid gland because of a worrisome nodule. The pathologist would confirm that the nodule was not cancer, but instead was from the benign disease of Hashimoto's Thyroiditis. In recent years the development of an easily available lab test for thyroid antibodies has confirmed that Hashimoto's is widespread.

Hashimoto's typically produces a confusing picture of both hyperthyroid and hypothyroid symptoms. One day you can be anxious with heart palpitations, and the next you may be so fatigued you can't even move. Typically, there is some weight gain. One of the most common presenting symptoms in my practice is myalgia. The problem in Hashimoto's is that the immune system has developed antibodies against both the thyroid gland itself and the thyroid hormones. When the immune processes are balanced, the person may have little in the way of symptoms. When the balance is toward the side of thyroid gland destruction, excess thyroid hormones will be released into the bloodstream and the person will appear to be hyperthyroid. When the balance is toward the side of the destruction of thyroid hormones, not enough hormones will get to the cells that need it for normal metabolic function. The person will effectively be hypothyroid. The balance between the two destructive processes can vary over time. Therefore, the symptoms also vary. Since myalgia can be present in both states, muscle pain is a relatively uniform symptom. In order to prevent the immune system from seeing the thyroid gland we often prescribe thyroid hormone. This suppresses thyroid hormone production and therefore the immune system does not see the thyroid gland. At the same time, sufficient levels of thyroid hormone can be built up in the blood to override the destruction of thyroid hormone by the immune system. I tend to prescribe Armour thyroid because it is taken from beef and pork thyroids. It is not identical to the thyroid hormone produced by our bodies, although it is close enough to ours to work. The *Levothyroxin* commonly prescribed by doctors for hypothyroid is bioidentical to that produced by our bodies and so can be more readily attacked by the immune system in Hashimoto's. Using prescribed thyroid hormone at a proper level seems to block the myalgic symptoms of the disease. Hashimoto's is a genetic disease, so it frequently runs in families. The majority of my Hashimoto's patients report that they have relatives who also have thyroid problems. Hashimoto's is more common in women than men, although it can be present in either sex.

Diabetes can also produce myalgia although it does not in every case. When the blood sugar is high for a long time it can produce a myalgic pain syndrome. This may be the result of direct activation of the pain nerves rather than from a metabolic problem of the muscles. However, glycosylation of muscle proteins may also play a role. Remember the active elements of muscle are protein as is fascia. Glycosylation will stiffen all protein. With decreased flexibility may come decreased mobility and increased pain.

Although it is rare, hyperactivity of the parathyroid gland can produce persistent muscle pain. The parathyroid gland manages calcium intake, storage in the bones and use in the body. Parathyroid tumors can cause blood levels of calcium to increase dramatically. High calcium levels result in persistent activation of all muscles, with increased and persistent tension, and muscle spasms resulting in pain throughout the muscle mass of the body. Correction of the elevated calcium levels results in normalization of muscle activity and resolution of myalgia.

MYALGIA AND PRESCRIPTION MEDICATIONS

Another major cause of muscle pain is prescription medication. Probably the most common prescription medications known to produce myalgia are statins. The statins include *lovastatin* (Mevacor), *simvastatin* (Zocor), *fluvastatin* (Lescol), *atorvastatin* (Lipitor), and *rosuvastatin* (Crestor). Together these medications all significantly lower cholesterol by blocking its production in the liver. The statins have been credited with a major reduction in the complications of vascular disease particularly in the heart. Although all these medications are known to have major, if rare side effects, such as the destruction of muscles (*rabdomyolysis*) and resulting kidney failure, these side effects are rare enough that the cost-benefit ratio is considered to fall almost totally to the side of the benefits. Therefore, many physicians tend to prescribe these medications freely. The makers of Crestor have recently even been able to gain approval of its prescription for those whose cholesterol levels are normal but have increased risk of heart disease for other reasons.

However, the statins have a dark side that is rarely considered by doctors and the drug companies. In addition to blocking production of cholesterol in the liver, they also block production of an enzyme called ubiquinone throughout the body. Ubiquinone is also known as Coenzyme Q10 or CoQ10. CoQ10 is an enzyme used by the mitochondria in all cells to change ADP to ATP. Essentially ATP is the energy molecule used to drive most of the metabolic functions in the cell. Most body cells can use alternative pathways to produce ATP. However, in neurons and muscle cells the CoQ10 energy pathway is required. As we age CoQ10 production naturally declines. The statin caused decline multiplies this natural process. Over time blocking CoQ10 production can result in lower-than-normal ATP in brain, nerves, and muscle cells. Decreased ATP seems to produce both brain fog and myalgia.

The amount of muscle pain produced by the statins varies. In some people myalgia is mild and merely irritating. I have been on statins for many years. My total cholesterol has always been normal but my good cholesterol was somewhat low and I did have a heart attack from stress in my early 50s. Given these facts the cardiologist had convinced me of the need to manage my cholesterol. At one point about 10 years ago, I switched from a low dose of Zocor to a similar dose of Crestor. Crestor is significantly more potent than Zocor on a milligram for milligram basis. About three months later I developed searing pain in my arms. It felt like a hot poker was being jammed along the length of all my muscles of both arms. The pain in my arms was bad enough that I began to worry that I would no longer be able to work as a manual medicine doctor. Nothing I took seemed to decrease the pain. After four weeks of wracking my brain, I began to wonder if this was the myalgia that my patients sometimes complained of from the statins. I finally realized that this horrid pain had begun shortly after I had changed to the new, more potent statin. So, I stopped taking it. Two weeks later the pain was gone.

I wasn't sure that in fact the statin was the culprit, although it seemed likely. So, I took the Crestor again. Within three days the searing pain in my arms was back. Once again, I stopped taking the Crestor. I ran the tests on myself to be sure that this wasn't *rabdomyolysis* (a rare complication of statins). After several weeks the pain had fully resolved. Since I had no problem taking Zocor before, I began taking it again. Unfortunately, once again I began to experience myalgia, although at a mild level.

Because the myalgic side effect of the statins was so apparent to me, I began to research what it was the statins were doing to cause such pain. It was easy to find information on the statin effect on CoQ10 production on the internet. In fact, the first reported research on the effect was published in a major medical journal in 1992. The information suggested that taking

CoQ10 on a daily basis would prevent the myalgia side effect. Over the years I have found that the proper dose to adequately prevent CoQ10 from dropping to levels that could produce myalgia is 200 to 400 mg per day. There is a newer formulation of ubiquinone called ubiquinol that is more easily absorbed. By taking 200 mg of CoQ10 a day I was able to return to taking Zocor without developing myalgia.

Many of my patients are over the age of 70. Many of these older patients come to see me for the first time with multiple complaints: back pain, neck pain, arthritis, and frequently, myalgia. Part of my intake questioning includes a cardiac history, cholesterol levels and medications. If they are on a statin, I always suggest they add CoQ10 to their regime to prevent side effects. Many of my older patients had been on statins before for their high cholesterol but stopped taking them because of myalgia. Since the data supporting use of statins for cardiovascular disease and elevated cholesterol is pretty convincing for people under the age of 80, I always suggest they give the statin another try but supplement it with 200 to 400 mg daily of CoQ10.

It was a little more work to discover that the drug companies had already taken out patents on the combination of their statin plus CoQ10. This told me they were aware of the relationship between their medications and this significant, although not life-threatening, side effect. Instead, they continue to minimize the CoQ10 problem and emphasize the beneficial effects of their medications. Because the drug companies have publicly ignored the CoQ10 problem, many doctors remain unaware.

Several other classes of medication have been implicated in lowering CoQ10 production. Prescription drugs known to lower CoQ10 include medicines used for managing cardiac disease and high blood pressure, including beta blockers Lopressor and Atenolol, the anti-hypertension drug Clonidine, tricyclic antidepressants such as Elavil (*amitriptyline*) and Tofranil (*imipramine*), the anti-psychotic drug Haloperidol, and diabetic sulfonylurea drugs such as Glucotrol (*glipizide*) and Micronase (*glyburide*). Although not clearly implicated in myalgic syndrome, all of these drugs can produce fatigue and leg pain and weakness as side effects. This would be consistent with an effect on lowering CoQ10 production. It could very well be that these various types of medications might also have an additive effect when it comes to the lowering of CoQ10, thereby worsening side effects of the statins.

CHAPTER 10
Posture

The position of our bodies as we stand, walk and sit is incredibly important in our body health. Posture can affect how efficiently our body operates in the world. Good posture is balanced and energy efficient. Bad posture inevitably requires more energy to do anything. Likewise with good posture we are comfortable. Bad posture results in discomfort and sometimes even pain.

When we stand and sit erect, our chest wall can fully expand and then relax allowing for a full deep breath. If we slump forward the diaphragm is crowded by our abdominal organs and cannot make a full piston movement in the chest. Our ribs are too close together along the front of our chest, limiting their natural movement. The end result of the slumped position: shallow breathing and little reserve capacity for when we need more oxygen and to blow off carbon dioxide.

As implied with breathing, slumping forward or slouching also crowds the organs in our abdomen. To some extent these organs can push forward because the abdominal wall is flexible and made only of muscle. However, poor posture has bad effects on digestion as well as decreasing the circulation of blood to and from our legs.

Walking and standing can be seriously compromised by poor posture. For instance, if the head and shoulders are slumped forward, they are in front of the normal center of gravity. When this occurs, the natural tendency is to fall forward. To prevent falling forward the back muscles have to work overtime, causing pain and fatigue. Walking is more difficult because balance is compromised, and each step becomes an act of falling forward and then catching the body's weight on the leg that is moving to the front.

AGING AND SLUMPING

Years ago, there was a TV skit involving a little old man played by Arte Johnson. The character would stand with his head thrust forward, shoulders and upper back rounded, and hips thrust forward. The character would shuffle rather than walk. The character's balance was so bad that he would fall off a tricycle. Years later, when asked how the character evolved, Arte Johnson said that he had seen old men and women who were like that but didn't understand until someone told him that their cataracts meant that seeing the world was like looking through glasses smeared with Vaseline. A method actor, Johnson tried the glasses and quickly realized that he couldn't see much beyond his feet. As a result, with the glasses he unconsciously adopted a head-forward and facing-down posture. He reasoned that gravity would then pull down on his head and neck. This would then round his shoulders and upper back. Standing and walking in this position was very unstable with a tendency to fall forward. To compensate he thrust his hips forward. In this position he was a bit more stable, but he could now walk only with short shuffling steps. The evolution of the little old man was complete.

Although the majority of older people with cataracts have them surgically corrected in this day and age, we still see many seniors with moderate to severe forward bending of the upper back. Sometimes this is due to compression fractures of the vertebral bodies. Osteoporosis in both males and females weakens the bone. Falls or other incidents forcefully pressing the vertebrae together can cause partial collapse of the vertebral bodies. In most cases the front of the vertebra body collapses more than the back giving it a wedge profile as seen from the side. One vertebra compression fracture probably won't affect posture very much. However, three or more generally leads to a strong forward bending of the spine. This is termed *kyphosis*. Kyphosis throws the head, neck and shoulders forward of the pelvis. The posture problems mimicked by the little old man character are likely to follow.

HEAD FORWARD

More common is the development of a posture problem that can be termed "head forward." The head is thrust forward. Commonly, the neck has a greater curve, so the face continues to point forward. Prominence develops at the base of the neck where it joins the back and shoulders. At its worst we call this prominence a dowager's hump. Some people begin to show signs of this in their 40s. It becomes increasingly common as people age.

Sometimes this develops as the result of trauma. One of my patients was a gentleman in his mid-70s. Ten years before he came to see me, he had been in a motor vehicle accident that involved severe front-to-back movement of his head and neck. This is termed whiplash. He did nothing about it for a few months. When it became clear to him and his wife that the new exaggerated forward thrust of his neck was not improving, he went to a spine surgeon. The surgeon told them that there were no fractures. The only thing the surgeon could suggest was a surgical fusion of his neck. Needless to say, they were shocked. The idea of losing mobility in his neck was unthinkable. They did agree to physical therapy. Unfortunately, this had little effect. By the time this patient came to see me 10 years later, his neck was held at about 90 degrees from the rest of his spine. The muscles at the back of his neck had become weak and thin with atrophy. To hold a conversation while erect he had to turn his head to the side in order to see who he was talking to. I wish I could say that I was successful in helping him recover. We did get some improvement in muscle tone and his neck was beginning to show a less pronounced forward thrust, but treating other disease processes became the priority and he stopped coming to see me.

Rarely is neck muscle atrophy so pronounced. However, if a person has been operating with a head-forward neck position for a long time, there is always some atrophy of the posterior neck muscles that must be overcome.

A more common cause of the head-forward neck position is the tendency to stand and sit with our shoulders rounded and our spine slumped. There was a time when the cultural norm was to correct young people who showed such a posture. Beginning in the 1950s, however, youthful rebellion overcame societal norms, except in the military. When I first started practice, I noticed the slumped posture more in females than males. Over the years I have come to realize that this problem affects both sexes and is an increasing problem as people age.

Part of the problem with the head-forward neck posture starts with the mechanics of the shoulder and arms. When we sit with our hands palm down on our legs, the shoulders are rolled forward and inward. It requires no effort to bend the head down and forward. In fact, it is extremely easy to assume the slumped head-forward position. The muscles at the back of the neck that attach to the wing bones or scapula are termed the trapezius. If the shoulders are rolled forward and inward the trapezius muscles have to relax.

On the other hand, if we sit with our hand palms facing upward the shoulders are rotated outward and backward. This causes tightening of the back muscles including the trapezius. Bending the head and neck forward actually requires effort. As a result, the palms-up position naturally keeps the head up with our ears in a vertical line with the sacrum.

The same logic applies when standing or walking. If we stand or walk with our arms at our sides but palms facing backward, the head and neck naturally fall forward. Our ears line up with our toes, not our heels. Over time this head forward position will result in rounded shoulders and possibly the development of a hump in the spine below the base of the neck. We do not need to stand or walk with our palms forward which is very awkward. A more reasonable standing and walking posture is found in the military stance. In the military stance our palms face our legs with the thumbs forward. In this posture the shoulders will be rotated lateral enough that the neck is naturally carried erect. Changing this habitual bad posture can be quite a challenge but the results are well worth it.

COMPUTER POSTURE

One of the incredibly strong influences on bad posture in our society is working with computers. In fact, computer-related injuries are some of the most common causes of workman's compensation claims in the United States. Much of the problem stems from improper relationships between our sitting, the keyboard and mouse, the placement of the computer monitor(s) and in some cases the placement of material we might be working from. If the keyboard is too high, as often is the case when we set it on the desk or tabletop, our arms, elbows and wrists must be actively held up. If we do not face the monitor with our body, we must hold our neck rotated to the side for prolonged periods. If we sit slouched in the chair, we force exaggerated abnormal curves in our neck, back and pelvis. If the monitor is too low or too high, we end up bending our neck forward or back in order to see. If the material we are working from is to one side, we must frequently move our head and neck on a diagonal as we move from the material to the screen and back again. Think about what this may be doing to you over an hour. A lot of damage can be done just in the course of a typical eight-hour workday.

There are two fundamental ways to improve the situation. The first is to institute what is termed proper computer ergonomics. The ideal position is to sit upright in your chair. Both feet should be on the floor. The hips and knees are at 90 degrees and the spine is erect. The computer screen is directly in front of your eyes without having to bend your neck. Plant your elbows at your sides. The keyboard should be positioned so that the elbows are at 90 degrees or a little less and the wrists should be resting on a supporting surface and approximately straight. Any material you are working from should be directly below the screen or to either side of the screen. If your computer workspace conforms to these standards, you are much less likely to suffer neck, back or arm problems.

A reasonable alternative for those working at computers is the standing desk. Although these are generally configured to ergonometric standards, there is some recent indication that standing all day is a potential cause of vascular disease. So ideally one would have a desk that can shift from sitting to standing and back with little effort, allowing the person to spend part of the day sitting and part standing.

The final computer-related posture issue is the increasingly popular laptop. A handy combination of CPU, keyboard, trackpad and monitor in one portable device, the laptop seems to be a good answer to many of our needs. However, working with a laptop is an ergonometric nightmare. Either the keyboard is too high or the screen is too low. Either we are lifting our arms and shoulders or bending our necks forward for too long. Many people who do a lot of computer work with a laptop are suffering from the pain and restrictions of neck motion seen in the neck-forward position. We probably cannot avoid these issues when traveling, but we can at home. Most laptops have some means of attaching a separate monitor, mouse and keyboard. If we use the laptop mostly as a CPU while at home and set the monitor and keyboard up in an ergonometric position, we will be much less likely to suffer musculoskeletal pain and restriction from working with our laptop computers.

ARTHRITIS

As we age most of us develop some degree of osteoarthritis of the spine. That can lead to stiffening of the spine. Most spinal flexibility is in the neck, the upper back at the level of the scapula or wing bones and in the lower back, or lumbar spine. Frequently osteoarthritis develops first in the lower or lumbar spine. Presumably this is because there are no ribs in the lumbar spine to help carry the load transmitted from the upper body. As the spine stiffens with age and arthritis, the most frequent limitations are in forward bending at the lower back. When an older person needs to bend forward, there is a tendency for more of the forward bending to involve the top part of the upper back and less of the lower spine. This can cause significant although transient abnormal posture when the older, arthritic person tries to bend forward.

SCOLIOSIS

Scoliosis is a term referring to a sideways curve of the spine. It actually has three different presentations and outcomes depending on when it starts, how bad it is, how long it has been present and which areas of the spine are involved. Scoliosis can be seen in the cervical, thoracic and lumbar spine. Often the upper sideways curves are partly in compensation to similar curves lower in the spine. Scoliosis is never normal.

The simplest, most common and most easily treated form is medically termed idiopathic scoliosis. It generally develops when we are adults. It frequently is the result of a minor trauma that does not involve any fractures, like a fall or stepping down a step unexpectedly. One hip is higher than the other and we see a functional short leg. The sideways curve is generally pretty minor, measured at 7 degrees or less. This type of scoliosis is typically limited to the low back or lumbar spine. Although the curvature can be seen on X-rays, there are no bony deformities. As long as it has not been present for a long time, treating the low back and pelvis will correct this type of scoliosis. Treatment by an osteopath or physical therapist is generally effective. Self-treatment may also help (see chapters on Helping the Low Back and Helping the Pelvis).

If idiopathic scoliosis of the low back has been present for a long time, there are a couple of complications that might prevent its successful resolution. One that is seen quite frequently when an idiopathic scoliosis has been present more than a year or two, is a compensating curve in the spine above the low back. If the low back is curved to the right, the upper back may become curved to the left. The other factor which is more concerning is when the back muscles around the scoliosis begin changing.

Typically, the muscles on the outside of the curve become stronger and more massive and muscles on the inside of the curve become weaker and begin to atrophy. If the curve has been present for years, aging and gravity may cause a gradual increase of the curve as the spine collapses toward the inside of the curve. The only successful treatment is to do exercises that unload the muscles on the strong side while exercising the weak muscle on the inside of the curve.

Sometimes fractures of the spine will produce scoliosis. If a compression fracture is greater on one side of the vertebra body, it will be wedged causing the spine above the fracture to bend to the side. Sometimes the facets on one side of the spine will fracture causing the spine at that level to rotate and bend to the side. In both cases scoliosis is not able to be treated, though strengthening the abdominal and back muscles may prevent further deterioration.

Finally, we come to infantile or childhood progressive scoliosis. While we do not know what causes the problem to develop, the curves are generally large (more than 27 degrees), and the disease involves steady worsening of scoliosis. Attempts to put the child in body braces are sometimes successful in arresting the collapse of the spinal sideways curves. However, the only definitive answer we have at this time is surgery fusing the spine in a straight configuration with rods.

CHRONIC STRUCTURAL IMBALANCE

A new development from Europe seems to provide an additional perspective and promise for those with chronic low back and pelvic pain. Part of this idea was discussed previously in looking at the effect of persistent muscle imbalance on developing a form of chronic pain. However, there is an additional factor that can come out of muscle inactivation and atrophy. This additional perspective comes from the work of Andry Vleeming, Ph.D., a Dutch rehabilitation physiologist.

First, during any movement involving the legs, hips, pelvis and low back a complex set of muscles is activated. Although American modeling of abnormal posture and movement for rehabilitation typically focuses on single joints, tendons, or ligaments, Vleeming's model suggests that any movement in the low back, pelvis, hips and legs involves a complex interaction of many muscles and joints, more like a big band or orchestra.

For the most part these movements are not under conscious control, even though the process may be consciously activated. Instead, the cerebellum, brainstem and spinal cord coordinate the patterns of muscle activation and inactivation that allow us to stand, sit, walk, bend or stoop. The actual sequence that determines which muscles activate when and for how long is driven by motor programs in the cerebellum. These are modified based on feedback from our skin and proprioceptors in the muscles, tendons, ligaments and joints.

Vleeming suggests that one of the important processes common to standing, walking, bending, getting up and sitting down is what he terms "force closure" of the pelvis. This is the use of muscles to compress the pelvis and stabilize the lower spine and sacrum. Some of the muscles involved in "force closure" cannot be activated consciously, particularly some of the inner abdominal muscles such as the transversis abdominis, internal abdominal oblique and the multifidus muscles of the low back. Vleeming used needle electrodes in multiple abdominal, pelvic, lower back and leg muscles. He showed in normal subjects that these muscles are activated in particular sequences, sometimes simultaneously, sometimes at various points during the sequence. The pattern varied depending on the action but was similar across all the normal subjects. In particular he noted that the multifidus muscles of the low back and the transversis abdominis tend to be active most of the time during any activity involving the low back, hips, pelvis and legs.

In patients with chronic low back and pelvic pain, Vleeming found that there is a failure of some muscles that are normally involved in activation patterns. In particular he noted a lack of activation of the inner abdominal muscles like the transversis abdominis, internal abdominal oblique and the multifidus muscles of the low back. Other muscles might have been weakened, but it was rare for those that could be used voluntarily to be inactivated. Sometimes these more voluntary muscles might become tight or painful simply because they were now being used in an inappropriate manner or at the wrong time in the sequence. Frequently, he also found the same type of structural imbalances that osteopathic physicians have traditionally treated. However, correction of tight muscles and structural imbalances were not enough to provide permanent relief for these patients from their chronic pain.

Vleeming developed the hypothesis that inactivation of core muscles involved in force closure was the source of chronic pain in these patients. Many had been disabled by their pain for more than five years. He accepted that psychological issues related to chronic pain and persistent structural imbalances were contributing factors. However, the reason that correction of these factors did not relieve chronic pain was that force closure was failing. Failure of force closure was due to inactivation of some key muscles that should have been more or less chronically active. Vleeming hypothesized that the activation failure was triggered by trauma. As discussed earlier in this book, the trauma could be physical or conceivably psychological. It could have been due to an accident, or even from surgery itself. In some cases, he even found it in women who had given birth. Once some of these muscles were inactivated, however, no effort to restore normalcy was effective unless the inactive muscles could be restored to normal function.

CHAPTER 11
Low Back

Low back pain is one of the most common experiences of pain in our lives. There are those who suggest that much of our low back pain develops because of the intrinsic instability of our erect posture and standing and walking on only two legs. From my standpoint, I see several problems with that idea. First, we often spend most of our young lives with little back pain, if any. When it does occur among the young it is most often the result of significant trauma or abuse. Second, much of our long-term back pain seems to be associated with aging processes and damage. Finally, if there was something intrinsically unstable about our posture and how we get from one place to another, it is doubtful that we would have continued to exist as a species. There is little evidence that our ancestors fared poorly because they did not have chiropractors and other musculoskeletal practitioners around to manipulate their spines.

When pain does exist in the back, we tend to attribute most of it to problems in the spine. While a significant portion of this pain may be due to the spine, there are other structures which can contribute. The first is the sacrum, on which the spine rests. We should always remember that the muscles of the back, the muscles of the abdomen, and the contents of the abdomen, particularly the kidneys, can contribute significantly to low back pain.

STRUCTURE OF THE SPINE

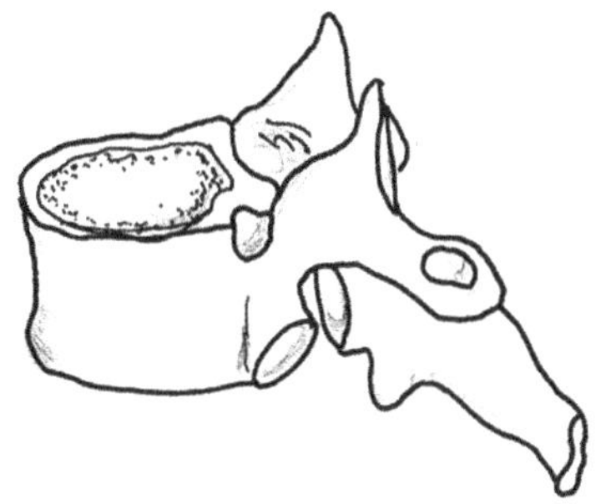

The spine consists of special bones, called vertebrae (Fig. 11-1). Each vertebra consists of a part like a hockey puck, the vertebral body. Between each vertebral body and those above and below are the discs. The disc is a gel-filled fibrous body that is flexible, as if it were made of rubber. This allows one vertebra to bend forward, backward and sideways on the vertebra below it. It also allows each vertebra to rotate to some degree relative to the neighboring vertebra. Behind the vertebral body is a bony ring that surrounds and protects the spinal cord. This is termed the neural arch. The inside of this bony ring is termed the spinal canal. The spinal cord and initial parts of the spinal nerves are encased inside this canal.

In order to keep the vertebrae from moving too far relative to each other, there are bony projections aligned vertically off the ring. The projections of two vertebrae mesh with each other to form joints. These are termed facet joints (or sometimes pars bones). Each vertebra in the upper back (the thoracic spine) and lower back (the lumbar spine) has four of these bony projections, two pointed up and two pointed down. The projections pointed up are oriented to slide against those pointed down on the upper vertebrae.

The general function of the facet joints is to keep the vertebrae from sliding too far forward or backward relative to its neighbors while allowing some rotation and forward and backward bending. Too much slippage to the front or back (termed *spondylolisthesis*) and the spinal cord and nerves will be crushed or even severed. Also, the facet joints keep each vertebra from rotating too far to the left or right at any one level. If we were able to rotate more than the facets allow, we could bruise or break the spinal cord and spinal nerves. Because of how these joints are aligned, movements on the diagonal are more likely to catch than movements such as bending forward (flexion) or backward (extension) or to each side (sometimes termed side-bending).

The major difference between the lower back, or lumbar spine, and the upper back, or thoracic spine, is the ribs. The upper back has twelve vertebrae with ribs attached on either side. This creates the barrel-like structure we term the chest since the ribs wrap around to the front where most of them attach to the breastbone, either directly or indirectly. The structure of the upper spine and ribs limits the range of motion of each vertebra. The lower back normally does not have any attached ribs.

The low back, or lumbar spine, has five vertebrae. They are numbered with the top lumbar vertebra labeled L1 and the bottom lumbar vertebra labeled L5. The lowest vertebra (L5) sits on the top of the sacrum. Because there are no ribs attached to the lumbar vertebrae, the lumbar spine is much more flexible than the upper back.

The basic structure of the spine, its vertebrae and discs allow us to stand upright with each vertebra bearing the weight of all the vertebrae above it. The structure of bodies, discs, the posterior ring or neural arch and the facets provides flexibility for the back and at the same time protection to both spinal cord and the nerves entering and leaving the spine. Unfortunately, this complex structure also sets us up for the possibility of pain.

STRUCTURAL BASIS OF LOW BACK PAIN

There are multiple ways in which the complex structure of the spine can fail to function normally and therefore produce pain. As suggested above, if there is too much slippage of one vertebra either forward or backward on the one below it, the nerves could be pinched as they exit or even inside the spinal canal. Sometimes a person is born without the facets that keep this from happening, particularly at the junction between the lowest lumbar vertebra (L5) and the top of the sacrum (S1). These people will have a natural tendency to develop low back pain.

Sometimes as we age the connective tissue that holds the facets to each other degenerates and the joints become too loose, also allowing front-to-back slippage. Sometimes a trauma will generate enough force that the facets will fracture. This can occur during a fall or even during an event that produces a lot of torque on our trunk, as sometimes happens in motor vehicle accidents. In each case, front-to-back slippage (spondylolisthesis) will be minor enough that it does not tear the nerves but can stress them or even compress them enough that we have pain. Sometimes it is not clear whether the pain is coming from the nerves in the spinal canal, nerves as they exit the spinal canal or nerve endings in the connective tissue around the spine because of the abnormal stresses.

As we age, gravity gradually causes compression of the discs between the vertebrae bodies. This is a major cause of the loss of height as we age. Other factors that can accelerate the effect of gravity include vertical forces through the spine while sitting, standing or jumping. As one of my mentors said years ago, "I seem to have lost three inches somewhere along the way and I can't seem to find them. I swear if I live long enough, I'll be a human pancake." Although a bit of an exaggeration, most of us lose height as we age due to the compression of our discs. Loss of disc height is accompanied by a loss of flexibility between the vertebrae. The facets are jammed together more than when we were young. The nerve outlets become smaller. Because the vertical height of the disc becomes shorter, the disc tends to bulge both along the outside of the spine and into the spinal canal. This too can contribute to narrowing of the nerve outlets.

As the discs compress, for the most part there is still enough space around the nerves to prevent them from being compressed. However, if we develop arthritic spurs on the edges of the vertebral bodies or on the facets, both of which are common, the amount of space for the nerve to exit is even smaller and the amount of space in the neural canal becomes smaller. This is termed *spinal stenosis.*

Collapsing discs, spinal arthritis and spinal stenosis do not cause pain on their own. Most of my older patients have one or more of these conditions and manage to go through long periods without back pain. They do frequently experience stiffness in the back, particularly after vigorous exercise or when first getting up in the morning. In general, their spine, particularly in the low back, is less flexible than when they were young. However, they do not have pain most of the time.

What produces pain in those with spinal disc degeneration, disc herniation, spinal arthritis and spinal stenosis? Some years ago, a study was done looking at the relationship between low back pain and herniated discs. For years the hypothesis was that a disc herniation would provoke low back pain and should therefore be surgically removed. Then a study examined the CT scans of the low back of a large group of 39-year-old males, some with low back pain and some without. The study showed that there was no relationship between having low back disk herniations and low back pain. Those with herniations were as likely to be pain-free as to have pain. Similarly, those with no disc herniations were equally likely to have low back pain or not.

Based on the experience of those who practice manual medicine, a primary source of back pain is the additional challenge caused by the development of a restriction in the normal mobility of the legs, hips, pelvis or spine. The restriction may be due to minor injury or trauma or just the chance events of life. No matter what our age, elements of our musculoskeletal system become slightly shifted and restricted in motion if we twist wrong, pick up something in the wrong way, trip or fall, step down a step unexpectedly, or habitually sit or stand with our weight poorly distributed. The osteopathic profession has termed these minor restrictions *somatic dysfunction*. Whether restriction is from arthritis, bursitis, muscle pain or somatic dysfunction, it doesn't just cause problems with the particular body part. Instead, as we've discussed previously, it develops a cascade of effects.

Suppose you go to build a house. Unfortunately, the contractor didn't take into account uneven firmness of the ground. After the foundation is poured and dries, it begins to settle on one side. It becomes unlevel. If the contractor continues to build the house on this crooked foundation as if it were straight and level, the house, too, will lean. The structural stresses on the house are abnormal from the beginning. This is what happened to the Leaning Tower of Pisa. Eventually the off-balance state will become so great that the house will fall over. If the contractor recognizes the unlevel nature of the foundation from the beginning an attempt can be made to correct for the crooked foundation by having the house lean the other way.

Our body is like the contractor who recognizes the out-of-balance nature and corrects it by having other parts of the body compensate. The compensations keep us from falling over and allow us to function. These compensations are active processes. They require unusual efforts by other parts of the body to perform normal functions. Remember the cases discussed earlier in which an unlevel pelvis produced an apparent leg length difference. Effectively this meant that when standing or sitting the pelvis was tilted toward the side of the short leg. To keep from falling over, the body tightens many muscles in the low back, buttocks and legs. It also tilts and rotates vertebrae in a way that compensates for the imbalance. The stresses of this process cause pain, not only in the hips and legs, but also in the spine. If this process lasts long enough, the compensation will extend all the way up to the neck and the person may even feel the pain more in the low back or neck than in the pelvis. Frequently compensation begins within the first few hours.

If the patient is older than 50 and also had some spinal arthritis and disc degeneration. the compensations produced in the spine might be enough to further close a nerve outlet. This would press on the nerve root and cause additional pain. Even worse, the tissues themselves would be slower to heal.

DUNLOP" SYNDROME

One of the classic causes of low back pain is the presence of a large abdomen. Years ago, when I was a medical student, I recall seeing an obese middle-aged patient who had severe low back pain. His X-rays and CT scans of the low back indicated a minor amount of lumbar spinal arthritis and disc degeneration. The neurosurgeon who was explaining the case to us did not feel that the patient's back pain was caused by his arthritis and disc degeneration. Instead, he stated that the patient's pain was being caused by Dunlop Syndrome. All of us looked confused. We had never heard of this particular disease. One of the students was brave enough to ask the physician what Dunlop syndrome was. The surgeon grinned at us and said, "Well, this patient's stomach has lapped over his belt. And like a pregnancy that never delivers, his stomach pulls strongly forward on his low back. Not even the strongest back muscles or best spinal health could prevent that forward pressure on the spine. The only thing that would help would be for the patient to lose weight."

The picture of that patient and the attending physician's description of "Dunlop Syndrome" have stuck with me all these years. When I have an overweight patient come in with a complaint of low back pain and a large or protuberant abdomen, I may tell them this story. No matter what else may be going on, losing weight and tightening the abdomen will help.

The issue of the protuberant abdomen and low back pain is part of a more general problem involving low back pain and muscle strength. Many of my patients ask me why their low back muscles were so weak. They assume that the pain in their low back comes from muscles that are not strong enough to support their low back.

There is more to this problem of low back pain than just the overweight abdomen pulling forward. The abdominal muscles in this case are typically weak and unable to contribute to normal back function. It is this issue of abdominal muscle weakness that is one of the major issues in low back pain.

If we look at the low back, upper back, chest and abdomen, we see a structure that looks like a flattened barrel. The upper back and chest together make up the thorax. The spine runs down the middle of the back. But the ribs attach to the spine and wrap around to the front where they attach to the sternum. Thus, the structure of the upper back and chest "barrel" is largely bone. Functionally, the weight of the arms, shoulders, head and neck and anything being carried on the head, shoulders, or arms is distributed down the front, sides and back of this bony barrel. The spine may bear a larger portion of this weight, but nowhere near all. Because a significant part of the upper body weight gets distributed away from the spine there is much less likelihood of pain and injury. In fact, the incidence of significant back pain is much less in the upper back than in the lower back.

In the lower back, the barrel that could take part of the load bearing down from the upper body is the muscular wall of the abdomen. With the exception of the spine the barrel is made up entirely of muscle. The abdominal muscles run vertically, horizontally and on the diagonal. They connect to the ribs, the pelvis and the spine. When these muscles are strong, they will pick up part of the load coming from the upper body and carry it down directly to the bones of the pelvis. When the abdominal muscles are weak or lax, most or the entire load from the upper body is funneled backward to the lumbar spine itself. Even without carrying a load, this may amount to between 35 and 40 percent of our body weight. If we are overweight this can produce upwards of 100 pounds of pressure down through the lumbar spine. Since the lumbar spine must also be flexible, the forces along the lumbar spine can be enormous.

Far from being weak, in most people the muscles of the low back are, in fact, quite strong even in the presence of low back pain. We do not need to strengthen them. However, if the abdominal muscles are weak, they will not be carrying their share of the load whether the abdomen is forward of the pelvis or not. Thus, when I discuss exercises for the low back, most of our exercises focus on the abdominal muscles, not on those of the lower back. In exercise physiology, physical therapy and physical training this is commonly termed "rebuilding the core."

PREGNANCY AND LOW BACK PAIN – A SPECIAL CASE

One special case of low back pain and the protruding abdomen is, of course, pregnancy. In this case, the structural problem is the same as the "Dunlop Syndrome." The stomach is protruding because the baby is growing. There is literally no place for the uterus and its contents to go but forward. After three months or so the belly is in front of the pelvis. In order to handle this weight cantilevered forward, the low back develops increased front-to-back curve (*lordosis*). Particularly if the new mother was not very athletic before pregnancy, or if she has gained excessive weight, she may experience significant low back pain whenever standing.

If the pregnant mother has low back pain it is often difficult to convince her that a solution to her pain could be found in exercise. Often, since the baby is crowding her other organs in the abdomen upward, it is harder to take deep breaths, and the downward pressure on the pelvis produces a pronounced waddle instead of her normal gait. None of this makes it easy to get the mother to exercise when she hasn't been doing it for a while, if ever.

In this situation manual medicine often can help the pregnant woman by removing any restrictions in the musculoskeletal system. Since such restrictions will add to the pain from the cantilevered position of her belly, manipulation seems to help. At least that has been the experience of osteopathic physicians over the past century. If and when the young mother does develop back pain, one effective means of relief is the "fallen chair position" discussed below. Lying down in the fallen chair position for even a few minutes a couple of times a day proves quite effective in relieving the low back pain of pregnancy.

The young woman who plans to get pregnant probably should start a program of at least modest exercise before she becomes pregnant. If she keeps exercising through the pregnancy, she will probably have an easier time with back pain through the pregnancy and an easier time with delivery. Such a program can be as simple as doing some abdominal muscle strengthening (see next chapter) and walking.

A HERNIATED DISC

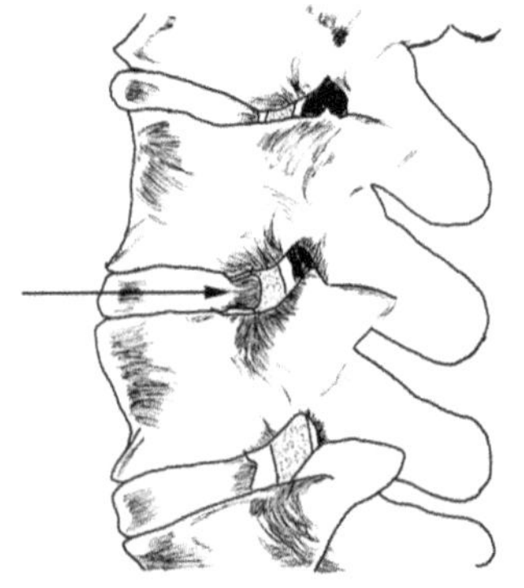

A spinal disc can also collapse due to tears in its outer fiber ring. This can allow the inner gel or nucleus of the disc to push out (Fig. 11-2). This is similar to what happens when you press on a tube of toothpaste. The tear in the disc wall and pushing out of the inner gel typically occurs when a sudden and unusual amount of force causes the disc to be compressed more than usual. This is termed a herniated disc.

Particularly if the herniation is inside the area of the neural canal, it can bulge backward and press on the spinal cord and/or the nerves as they leave the spine. Essentially this produces an acute form of spinal stenosis. It is not clear how much pain is produced by the actual tear itself. There are no nerves in the inner disc gel, so the pain is not from the gel itself. The disc wall has some pain nerves, but not a lot. It is assumed that most of the pain from a herniated disc occurs when the gel presses on the spinal cord or nerves in the neural canal or on the nerves as they leave the spine. The pattern of pain produced by a herniated disc will at times predict where the disc has herniated. Therefore, if the herniation is pressing on the nerves as they exit between the lowest lumbar vertebra (L5) and the top of the sacrum (S1) on the right, you may feel pain, numbness and tingling down the outside front of the right leg and into the top of the right foot.

However, not all disc herniations produce pain. Remember the herniated disc study discussed earlier. Half of the men in the study had low back pain and half did not. Radiological studies were then done on all of them, but the radiologists reading the studies had no idea who had low back pain. Equal numbers of those with and without pain were found to have no evidence of herniated discs. This is not so surprising since not everybody who has back pain has a herniated disc. What did surprise us was that equal numbers of those who had back pain and no back pain had a herniated disc. That is, the presence of herniated discs did not always produce pain.

In my practice I have seen and treated quite a few patients who were found to have herniated discs in the lumbar spine. Some of them were patients who came to me with known herniations but wanted to avoid surgery if possible. Some of them were patients who came to me with low back pain and were found on examination to have herniated discs, like one recent patient.

This patient was a 59-year-old man who had fallen while playing tennis. He came to see me on the advice of a friend. A new patient to my practice, he had developed severe low back pain with radiation into his left leg after the fall. He had never before had low back pain. He enjoyed good health and was visibly vigorous and well-muscled, although he came in bent over at the waist like a very old man.

As I examined him it quickly became apparent that he had a more significant injury than most of my patients. Although the skin sensation in both legs was the same, he had a numbing pain down the back and side of his left leg. The straight-leg-raising test was positive for his left leg. Fortunately, he had not lost control of either bowel or bladder, which would have been a medical emergency. He had sheared his left pelvis upward so that his left leg was shortened by ½ inch. He had a significant lumbosacral strain pattern indicating he had twisted as he fell.

I was convinced enough of the nature of his injury to order an MRI of his lumbar spine. Because it would take several days before the results would be available, I gave him a prescription for a few days' worth of prednisone and taught him a position he could get into that would relieve his pain. For lack of a formal name for this position, I will term it the "fallen chair" position (see next chapter). This position is well known in both surgical and osteopathic literature for relieving low back pain including that from herniated discs. Unfortunately, the relief lasts only as long as you are in the position.

The MRI showed what I suspected. My new patient had a herniated L5 disc. The herniation was toward the left side, pressing on the nerve as it exited the outlet. There was some swelling around the nerve indicating that the herniation was recent. There was only minor arthritis present and moderate disc degeneration throughout the lumbar spine.

The patient reported that he had about 50 percent improvement in his pain after his initial treatment and several days on prednisone. I found this encouraging. I offered to send him for a consultation with a back surgeon but suggested that we give a combined course of manual medicine and prednisone for about 20 days. He was agreeable, particularly since he had no wish to go through surgery. I cautioned him that if his pain got worse or if he lost control of bowel or bladder it should be considered a medical emergency and he should go immediately to the Emergency Room. Since any compressive forces affecting his spine might worsen the herniation, he was advised not to go to the gym or play golf or tennis for a few weeks.

Over the course of the next three weeks, he became progressively better. All of the restrictions in motion around his spine and pelvis resolved with manual medicine. The pain in his left leg disappeared as did his low back pain. He felt so much better he was pressing me to allow him to restart his exercise routine. Since I agree in general that exercise is important to help manage most forms of musculoskeletal pain, I had him start to exercise his legs in a swimming pool. From there he was quickly able to progress to riding a stationary bicycle and then walking. By six weeks after his injury, he was back to playing tennis without pain.

This patient's recovery was rapid but well within what I commonly see in my practice. In general, the available data from the back-surgery literature suggests that more than 80 percent of all acute disc herniations will resolve within a month without a need for surgery. Thus, the presence of a disc herniation should not be taken to mean that surgery is unavoidable. Surgery may be necessary but should be reserved until after more conservative measures have been tried, including just waiting it out.

SPINAL COMPRESSION FRACTURES

When the force that goes through the spine is sudden and strong it may fracture the body of a vertebra rather than blow out a disc. When the bones of the spine have become porous and brittle, such a fracture is an increased possibility particularly with a fall onto the buttocks or back. The fracture may be direct and vertical to the body of the vertebra. This will produce a general collapse. From the side, the body of the collapsed vertebra body looks rectangular but is much shorter than those above and below (fig. 11-3a). More commonly the force produces a collapse of the vertebra that is greater at the front surface of the vertebral body than the

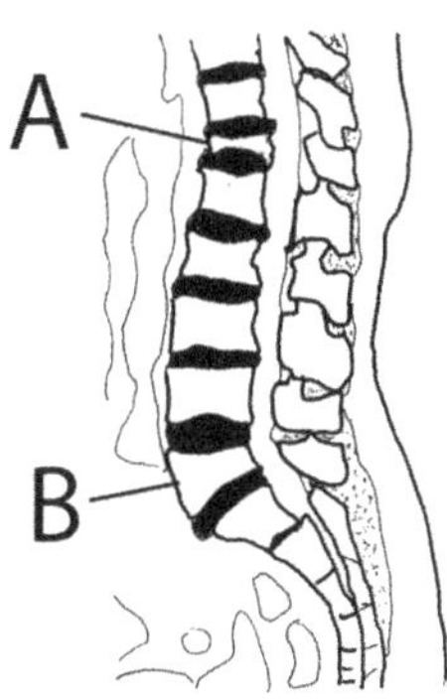

back. From the side this will make the vertebra look like a wedge (fig. 11-3b). Both forms of fracture are termed compression fractures.

All compression fractures of the vertebrae are very painful. Partly this is because the bone is broken and partly because the altered shape stresses neighboring tissues. Any movement of a broken bone is painful. Partly, the pain from a compression fracture is the result of the alteration of normal spinal mechanics and the resulting muscle activation to both compensate and splint around the fracture. And partly it is from the nerves to the connective tissue covering the bones, joints and discs. It is suspected that the compression fracture alters the nerve outlets, potentially compressing and damaging the spinal nerves.

Although most broken bones heal in about six weeks, spinal compression fractures typically take up to six months. Probably most of the delay in healing is because we must spend most of the day upright. Compression from the weight of the body above the fractured vertebra does not stop just because the vertebra is fractured. Unfortunately, we have no practical way to cast or immobilize the vertebra as we would a broken arm.

Years ago, we had virtually nothing to offer someone with a vertebral compression fracture except narcotics to deaden the pain. It was going to take six months or longer to heal no matter what. Then, in the middle 1990s, it was discovered that injecting the body of a fractured vertebra with "super glue" (*cyanoacrylic*) would stabilize the fractured elements. For the most part it would also eliminate the pain of the fracture almost as soon as it was injected. The original technique was called *vertebroplasty*. Unfortunately, when the super glue was injected, there was the possibility that some would leak out of the fractured bone. In those rare cases it could cause nerve damage, which, of course, would produce pain. Over the years, the technique has evolved to include an additional and important step. Now a small balloon is inserted into the fractured vertebra. Inflating the balloon with superglue keeps the super glue from leaking out of the vertebra. Inflating the balloon also tends to expand the bone so that it looks more normal. The process is termed *Kyphoplasty*. It is very effective in relieving pain from a vertebral compression fracture as long as the fracture is less than six months old. It does not, however, have any useful effect on fractures older than six months, probably because they have already healed.

LUMBAR SCOLIOSIS

The normal curve for the lumbar spine is bowed from front to back. The upper and lower ends of the lumbar spine (L1 and L5) are further back. The middle lumbar vertebra (L3) is more toward the front of the body. This bowing is termed *lordosis*. When there is little or no lumbar lordosis it is usually the result of trauma. The lumbar spine does not typically show any sideways curves. When sideways curves do exist, they are termed scoliosis (Fig. 11-4).

As previously discussed, if the sideways curves of the spine are very pronounced, they are unstable and may become progressively worse. The most severe form is infantile scoliosis which occurs in childhood or the early teenage years. As discussed in the last chapter, stabilizing infantile scoliosis requires body casts, exercise, and surgical rodding and fusion. Similar high-grade lumbar scoliosis can sometimes be seen in older adults after years of gravity have exaggerated their once minor scoliosis into high-grade scoliosis. Unfortunately, severe adult lumbar scoliosis is rarely treated surgically.

Much more common are shallow sideways curves of the lumbar spine. Although teachers and school nurses are taught to look for all sideways curves of the spine, most are minor and not surgical. In my experience, most lumbar scoliotic curves are part of a pattern of compensation for either an anatomical short leg or some form of strain pattern involving the pelvis and low back. To examine the spine for such a curve is simple. Have the person to be checked stand in front of you. Look at the spine with the person standing erect. If there is a side-to-side curve, how easy is it to see? Now have them bend forward at the waist. As they bend forward, look at the spine. If there is no side-to-side curve, no scoliosis is present. If the curve is easily visible in both positions and one side of the back or shoulder seems to stick backward, the scoliosis will need to be evaluated by a physician. If the curve is small, it would probably help to have the spine and pelvis treated by someone who practices manual medicine.

It is not uncommon for me to see people with mild lumbar scoliotic curves. Often, they are like a 14-year-old young woman brought to me by her mother. She was very active in sports: gymnastics, basketball and bicycle riding. Her gym teacher had commented to the mother that she had scoliosis and should be seen by a physician. She had been taken to an orthopedic surgeon who told her mother that the scoliosis was slight and most likely not progressive or requiring surgery. The mother was instructed to watch her daughter. If there was any sign that the curve was getting worse, she was to bring her back. Instead, the mother brought her daughter to see me.

This new young patient had a very minor but noticeable sideways "S" curve to her spine involving both the upper and lower spine. It was more pronounced in the lumbar spine but was still mild. I also evaluated her for other signs of musculoskeletal restriction. What I found was that she had rotated and restricted both sides of her pelvis effectively giving her a 5/8-inch leg length difference. As soon as that and some spinal compensations were treated with manipulative medicine, the scoliotic curves in her spine disappeared. She has been fine since.

SCIATICA AND PINCHED NERVES

Frequently when patients come to see me, they complain about having "sciatica" or a problem with their sciatic nerve. The term has entered the common language to mean anything from a pain that goes down the leg in some fashion to pain in one buttock. In medical terms sciatica is a pain that goes down the back of the leg due to compression of the sciatic nerve.

The sciatic nerve is a large nerve that connects to most of the muscles and skin of the leg. It is made of several nerve roots that exit from the lumbar spine and collect together in front of the sacrum. The sciatic nerve exits the pelvis behind the hip joint. It then goes down the back outside part of the thigh (see Chapter 13, fig 13-2). True sciatica, as defined by medical professionals, involves compression of one or more of those nerve roots as they exit the spine. Typical sciatic pain runs from the lower buttock down the back of the thigh and into part of or the whole lower leg and foot.

Pain that is confined to the buttock is generally muscular and not due to compression of part of the sciatic nerve. However, the sciatic nerve does come out of the pelvis between several of the buttock muscles. If buttock muscles are having spasms, they can pinch or compress the sciatic nerve and produce a pain down the back of the leg that looks like the sciatica that comes from nerve compression at the spine. Often it takes a physician to be able to tell the difference. The sciatica caused by muscle spasms in the buttock is much easier to treat.

Pain down the side of the thigh is typically not from sciatic nerve compression. It is most likely due to excessive tension in the thick tissue band that runs from the pelvic crest down to the knee, termed the iliotibial band or IT band (Fig. 11-5). That can occur as part of the body's attempt to compensate for an imbalance in the legs or pelvis. It can also occur as a result of bursitis over the outside bony part of the upper thigh bone (termed the greater trochanter of the femur). In either case it does not result from a pinched nerve.

If you have pain, numbness or tingling down the front of the thigh it is most likely from the pinching of a sensory nerve in the groin. I experienced this problem after the cardiologist catheterized my heart. The nerve that comes from the skin on the front of the thigh goes upward into the groin before going in toward the spinal cord. It runs right next to the artery providing blood to the leg. Heart catheterization is usually done through this femoral artery. Heart catheterization sometimes pinches or damages the nerve running next to it. This damage is common enough to have its own name: *meralgia paresthetica*.

Finally, I have had patients who reported what they termed "sciatica" but when questioned further, reported that the pain was in their groin. If it also involves the flank on the same side, it is from spasm of an abdominal muscle termed the external abdominal oblique. If it involves the upper front of the thigh just below the pubic bone, it is probably from a strain or pull of a short muscle termed pectineus. This site of muscle spasm is often termed a groin pull and is common in athletes. If it involves the muscles on the front of the thigh, the quadriceps, it will also be associated with difficulty fully bending the knee. In all these cases the groin pain is not sciatic and does not normally involve a pinched nerve.

A final form of leg pain that results from a pinched nerve occurs because of restrictions on the lateral or outside part of the knee. The sciatic nerve as it crosses the lateral part of the knee is termed the peroneal nerve. If there is a restriction in the tissues on the lateral surface of the knee, the nerve can be pinched, causing pain, numbness, and/or tingling in the lower leg and foot. The abnormal feelings will not involve the upper leg and so is not really sciatica.

CHAPTER 12
Helping the Low Back

There are a number of exercises for low back pain. Three of these exercises address low back muscles directly. Each is based on the unique roles these three muscles seem to play in the generation or maintenance of low back pain. Muscle fatigue, imbalance and atrophy can cause low back pain independent of the mechanisms covered in the previous chapter. Most of the rest of the exercises recommended for managing low back pain focus on the abdominal muscles and on more general conditioning.

The "Fallen Chair" position for easing the low back: The "fallen chair" position is simple. It is very relaxing to the low back and, in most cases, will relieve low back pain at least for the period while you are on your back.

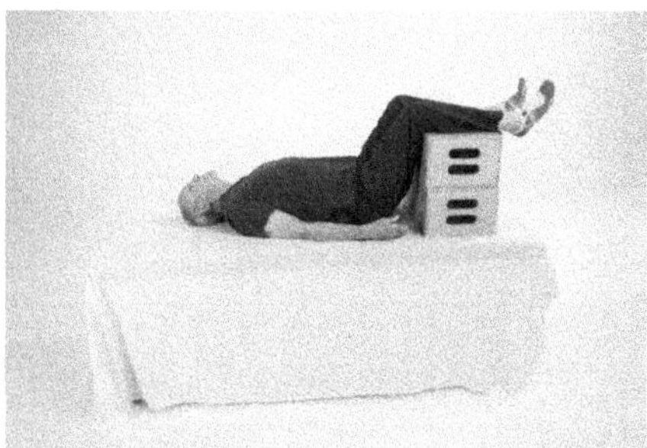

1. Lay on your back. It doesn't matter whether you lay on a bed or a firmer surface.
2. Bend your knees to about 90 degrees.
3. Put your feet up on a stool or hassock. This will bend your hips to about 90 degrees. (Fig. 12-1) You now look like a chair that has fallen over on its back.
4. Stay in this position between three and 20 minutes.
5. To get out of this position, roll over to your side. If you are on a bed allow your feet and calves to fall off the side of the bed.
6. Push up to the side with your arms so you are seated on the side of the bed.
7. If you are on the floor, roll over to your hands and knees. Use your hands and arms to push or pull yourself upright and then to a standing position.

FATIGUE IN THE QUADRATUS LUMBORUM

The Quadratus Lumborum is a muscle that runs from the bottom of the rib cage down to the crest of the pelvic bone. It is a flat muscle that is found about two to three inches to either side of the spine. Each muscle continues laterally to the outer edge of the back where it changes into the flank. The muscle is rectangular in shape. The Quadratus Lumborum acts primarily to stabilize the back as we walk and stand. It is more or less always active.

One of the unusual characteristics of the Quadratus Lumborum is that it has an unusually large number of muscle fibers that are termed slow twitch. Most skeletal muscles are made up of fast-twitch fibers. These fibers are good at rapid movement, but fatigue rapidly if asked to sustain their activity. Slow-twitch fibers, on the other hand, are not very quick in their action but are set up to act in a prolonged fashion. Therefore, they tend to play a major role in posture. Since Quadratus Lumborum has an unusually high percentage of slow-twitch fibers, it is assumed to have a large role in maintaining posture as well as in changing positions.

In low back injuries it is frequently the case that Quadratus Lumborum becomes inflamed. After the injury and inflammation heals, Quadratus Lumborum seems to fatigue easily. It acts as if many of its slow-twitch fibers have been replaced by fast-twitch fibers. It has been well-documented that rats, when subjected to prolonged gravitational stress (living in a centrifuge), change the muscle fiber composition of many of their leg muscles. Muscles that normally are entirely composed of fast-twitch fibers are found to have large numbers of slow-twitch fibers. It appears that under a continuous load, fast-twitch fibers can change to look and act like slow-twitch fibers. Although the experimental data are less conclusive, there is evidence that when slow-twitch fibers are subjected to increased variable loads, they will switch to fast-twitch fibers. This seems to be the case with the Quadratus Lumborum.

Once a portion of the slow-twitch fibers in the Quadratus Lumborum change to the more easily fatigued fast-twitch fibers, the muscle itself has a harder time carrying its share of the postural load. It fatigues easily. When it becomes fatigued, the nociceptors within the muscle become active. In other words, you have an aching back.

When my patients are asked where their low back pain is, they often point to Quadratus Lumborum. Their history is often one of minor low-back injury, but with an inability to recover fully. Often, they report increased back pain with standing or sitting, but little pain if sitting with the back fully supported or if they are lying down.

A quick way to tell whether Quadratus Lumborum is fatiguing is to ask the patient to stand erect holding a one- or two-pound weight in the hand on the side of the low back pain. Even if there is no pain initially, within a minute or two the pain will appear in the low back. The muscle that was perhaps only mildly tender before now becomes very tender. If the patient sits in a chair with good back support, the pain will go away. The exercise to treat easy fatigability in Quadratus Lumborum is simple:

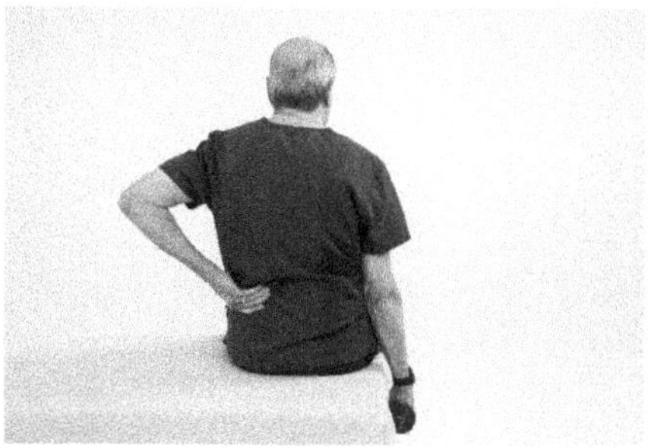

1. Sit in a chair. The back should not be supported. A weight of at least five pounds is in the hand opposite the Quadratus Lumborum to be treated.
2. The hand with the weight should be dangling at your side (Fig. 12-2). The weight will tend to cause you to bend towards its side.
3. Resist by sitting erect for at least two minutes. Initially you may feel the rapid fatigue of the muscle as a burning.
4. Over the period of a week build up to five minutes.
5. If the pain in your back has been on both sides, treat the other side in the same fashion.

As easy as this exercise seems, it may take a number of weeks, even months, before the Quadratus Lumborum returns to its normal ability to be active in both movement and posture. However, once it does, you may experience a significant reduction in your low back pain.

IMBALANCE IN LOW-BACK MUSCLES

Often when a scoliotic curve is present for any length of time, an imbalance will develop in the low-back muscles on both sides of the spine.

Remember, a scoliotic curve is one in which there is a sideways curve, like a bow. The muscles on the inside of the bow are shortened and those on the outside are lengthened. As long as this muscle imbalance has not been there so long that the muscles have atrophied and become fibrotic, we can have a significant effect on these imbalances. We have to stretch and at the same time strengthen the muscles on the inside of the bow and strengthen those on the outside of the bow. To stretch and strengthen the muscles on the inside of the bow, we need to use a weight that will tend to bend the spine toward the other side.

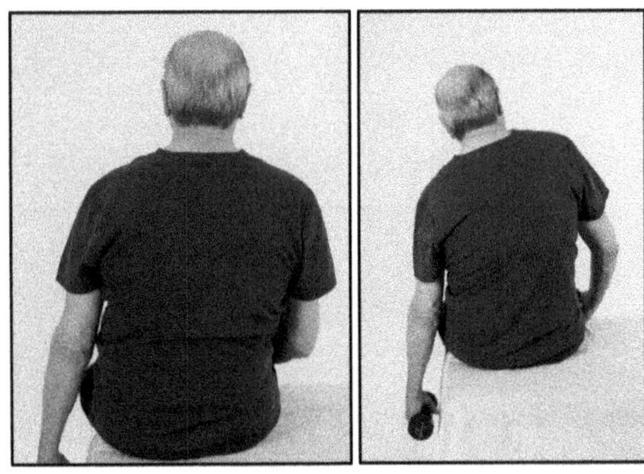

1. Sit on a chair.
2. Have a weight in the hand that is opposite the short side of the curve (Fig. 12-3a). It is best to use a five-pound weight, but you may have to start with less.
3. Let the weight pull the spine into a straighter position or even toward the opposite side (Fig. 12-3b).
4. Briefly and gently try to bend away from the weight.
5. Now again let the weight pull down on your arm, bending in the opposite direction. Repeat 20 times.

Now we can do a similar exercise to strengthen the muscles on the outside of the curve.

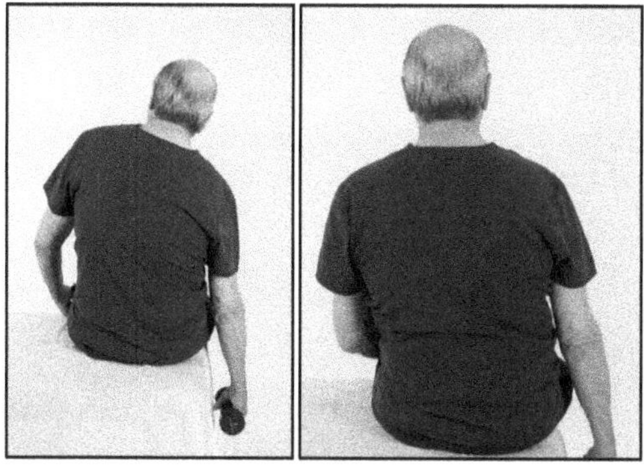

1. Transfer the weight to the hand on the short side of the curve (Fig. 12-3c).
2. Actively bend away from the short side of the curve (against the weight) (Fig. 12-3d) as many times as possible. The target is 10 repetitions.

Over time these combined exercises will help rebalance the muscles that have been supporting a mild scoliotic curve.

MUSCLE WEAKNESS IN THE MULTIFIDUS MUSCLE

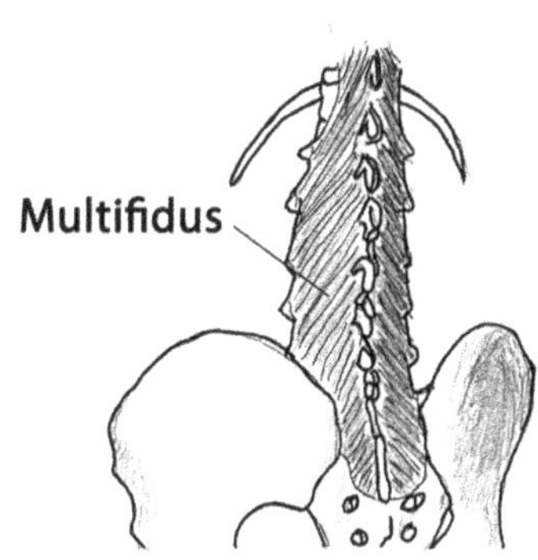

Remember Dr. Vleeming's suggestion that muscle atrophy and weakness are triggers for chronic back pain (Chapter 10). In the low back, the principal culprit identified by Dr. Vleeming is the multifidus muscle. This muscle is small, but because of its location at the base of the spine it plays a crucial role in maintaining balance of the spine on the sacrum. The multifidus muscles attach to the back of the lumbar spine and to the sacrum and pelvic bones (figure 12-4).

What Dr. Vleeming found is that after injury to the pelvis or lower back, the multifidus stops being active on one side of the spine or both. With inactivity comes weakness and pain whenever you sit upright or stand up. The pain can be very debilitating. In fact, most of Dr. Vleeming's recent work involved people with so much back pain that they were on disability. When he identified a patient with chronic low-back pain who showed signs of inactive multifidus muscles, he tried various methods of bringing them back to normal activity. Finally, he hit on a form of biofeedback that seemed to work well in restoring normal activity to the multifidus. When the multifidus became consistently active, the patient's back pains disappeared and they were able to get off of disability.

Unfortunately, it is not possible for us to actually identify whether an inactive multifidus muscle is responsible for at least part of our low-back pain on our own. That process requires either use of electrodes to identify muscle activity, or a physician who can do this by monitoring the muscle during a specific exercise that should activate it. If you have back pain because multifidus is not working properly, doing these exercises should help relieve the pain, perhaps permanently. Using the feedback activation exercises will do no harm if the muscles are functioning normally.

The multifidus feedback exercises are relatively simple. Pressure of your fingers on the weakened or inactive muscle is critical to get your body and brain to recognize that muscle and reintegrate it into normal activity. The position of your fingers should be on the multifidus muscles just next to the spinous processes at the lower back-hip junction as shown in (Fig. 12-3). The seated version is the easiest or beginning version:

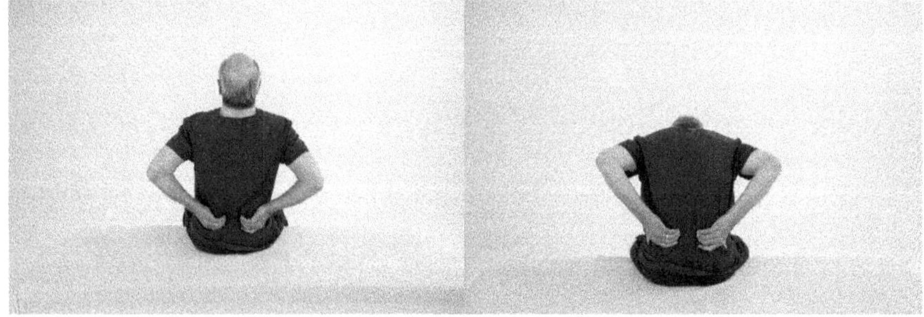

1. Sit straight on a chair with your back about a foot in front of the back of the chair.
2. Your fingers press firmly on the multifidus muscles to the right and left of your spine at the lower back-hip junction.
3. Bend back until your shoulders touch the chair back (figure 12-5a).
4. Now bend forward so your shoulders are over the middle of your thighs (figure 12-5b).
5. Repeat five to 10 times.

If you can do these easily, graduate to the prone version (lying on your stomach):

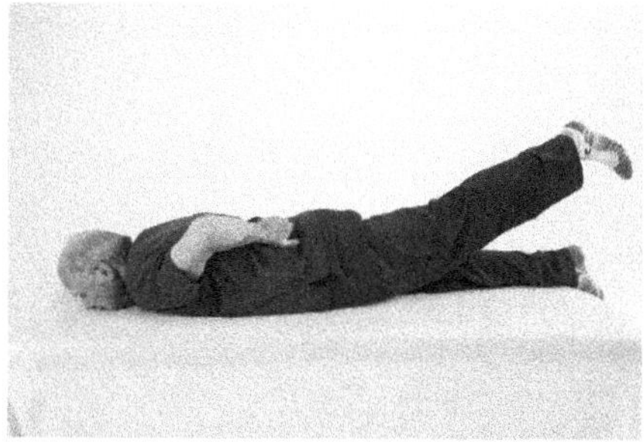

1. Lay on your stomach.
2. Fingers press the lower back-hip junction next to the right and left sides of the spine.
3. Lift the thigh and leg of one side backwards off the table (figure 12-6).
4. Now return it to the surface on which you are lying.
5. Repeat five to 10 times.
6. Do the same for the other side.

These muscles have been inactive for a long time. As a result, it is very likely that they will be sore as they are reactivated and brought into constant use. Remember that it is critical that you use your fingers to put pressure on the multifidus muscles as you are doing the exercises. The pressure from your fingers provides the feedback so that the body will begin to recognize the muscles and reintegrate them into normal patterns of use. Using the feedback activation exercises will do no harm if the muscles are functioning normally.

OTHER MUSCLES RELATED TO LOW-BACK PAIN

With a couple of exceptions, most exercises for low back pain that I recommend are not to strengthen the low back. This may seem paradoxical to most people who are used to the idea that you treat the area of injury. However, with a couple of significant exceptions covered above, most back pain does not arise from weakness or imbalance in the muscles of the low back.

Recall that we looked at the torso as being in the shape of a barrel. The upper back barrel used the rib cage to carry part of the weight away from the spine. For the lower back, the abdominal muscles must do the same. If abdominal muscles are weak or loose, or the belly simply extends forward of the front of the pelvis, the majority of the upper body weight will be concentrated in the spine itself. This tends to put too much pressure on a structure that is only a couple of inches in diameter and has to remain flexible.

In general walking, running, bicycle riding, swimming, dancing and other sports will help develop abdominal muscle strength. However, unless one is relatively slender and regularly active, it is rarely enough. Interestingly, the ripped abdominal muscles of the body builders aren't exactly what the doctor ordered either, even though we may think they look good. The most effective abdominal muscles are those that have endurance. We are really looking for the abdominal muscles to act more like postural muscles rather than to have that explosive, but short-acting, strength seen in washboard abs. Sit-ups performed slowly can produce this. Rapid sit-ups may be less effective in controlling back pain. To achieve the best strengthening from sit-ups it is better to place your hands on your chest rather than behind the neck because you don't want to pry your neck. Everything must be from the belly. Sit-ups performed with the hands behind the neck or head tend to overstress the neck and there is a tendency to tense the shoulders rather than work the abdominal muscles.

TRANSVERSUS ABDOMINIS FEEDBACK ACTIVATION

Transversus abdominis is a muscle that runs laterally across the abdomen. It is the deepest muscle layer in the abdominal wall. Dr. Vleeming identified this as another of the muscles that tends to drop out when there has been injury or trauma to the low back. Normally it acts in concert with the rectus abdominis and external abdominal oblique muscles to stabilize the barrel of the abdomen. When it is weak, it contributes to low back pain.

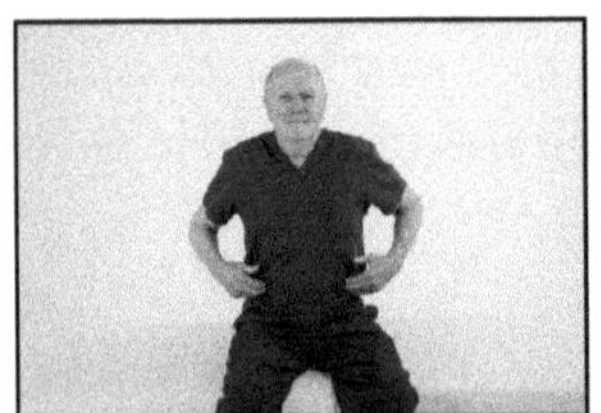 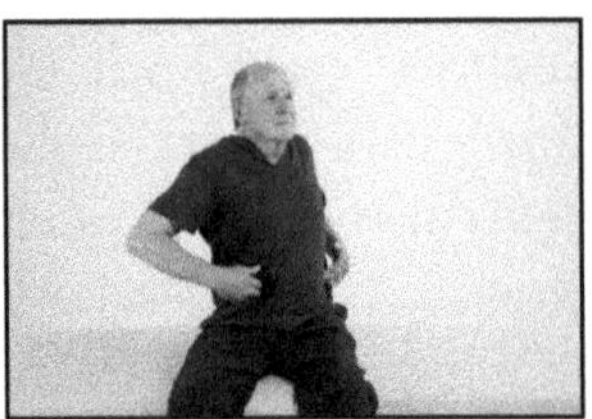 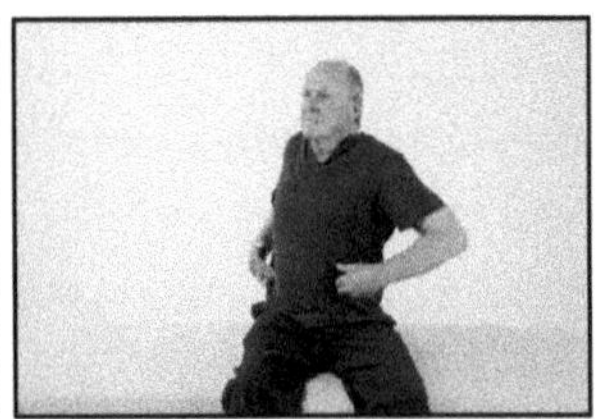

1. Sit on a chair.
2. Press the fingertips of both hands on the outside front of your stomach about three inches lateral to your belly button (Fig. 12-7a).
3. Rotate your shoulders (not your neck) to the left (Fig. 12-7b)
4. Then rotate all the way to the right (Fig. 12-7c).
5. Repeat five to 10 times.

STRETCHING AND RELAXING THE EXTERNAL ABDOMINAL OBLIQUE

The external abdominal oblique muscles run diagonally from the bottom of the rib cage in the back, sweeping around and down toward the front. The tendons of this flat muscle insert on the lateral hip crest and also sweep further forward ending on the tendon in the middle of the abdomen (linea alba) and on the pubic bone. The actual muscle fibers normally end above the front end of the hip crest, a projection termed the anterior superior iliac crest (ASIS). The bottom end of the external abdominal oblique muscle tendon gathers into a structure often called the inguinal ligament running between the ASIS and the pubic bone. If there is tension or long-term shortening of the external abdominal oblique muscle, there can be significant groin pain along with low back pain. It is rare for this muscle to become weak. Therefore, most of the management involves relaxing it when it is tight and provoking pain. If it is weak, it will be strengthened by rotating the trunk as is done with the exercise for Transversus abdominis discussed above.

To relax the external abdominal oblique muscles:

1. Lay on your back.
2. Bring the knee of the side you want to relax up to 90 degrees.
3. Let the leg fall toward the outside (see fig. 12-8).
4. Support the leg by holding it in place with your hand from the same side. Hold this position for two minutes.
5. If you need to relax the external abdominal oblique from both sides, you can do both at the same time.

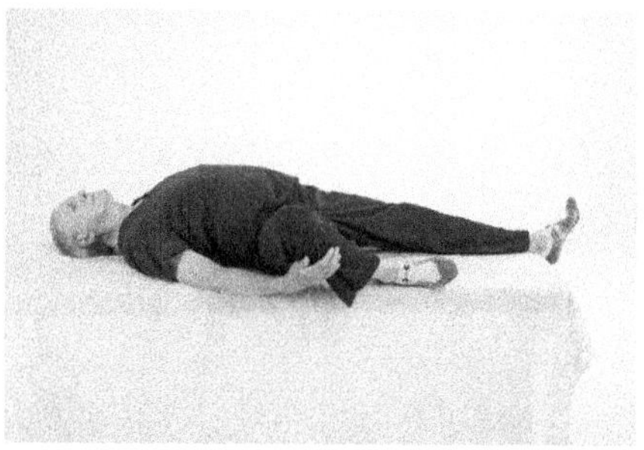

To stretch the external abdominal oblique muscle:

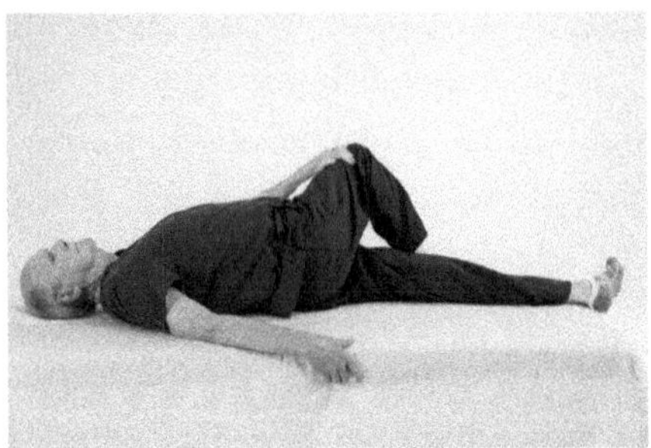

1. Lay on your back with both legs stretched out.
2. If you are trying to stretch the right external abdominal oblique muscle, bend your right leg.
3. Put your right foot next to the outside of your left leg. The best position would be with the right foot at about the middle of the left thigh (Fig. 12-9).
4. Place your left hand on the outside of your right thigh (Fig. 12-9).
5. Gently push against your left hand with the right thigh for three brief pulses. You do not need to push strongly with this move since the purpose is to inactivate the tight muscle.
6. Now press the right thigh more to the left with your left hand.

REBUILDING YOUR CORE

Over the years quite a number of exercises have been developed and promoted for rebuilding the abdominal or "core" muscles that have become weak with time and inattention. They range from sit-ups and crunches to twisting crunches to leg raises while hanging from a bar or parallel bars. Two that I have found particularly helpful are listed below.

THE "V" CRUNCH

A most effective exercise for building endurance muscles for the abdomen is one I learned in the martial arts. The two initial steps are later combined to produce a "v."

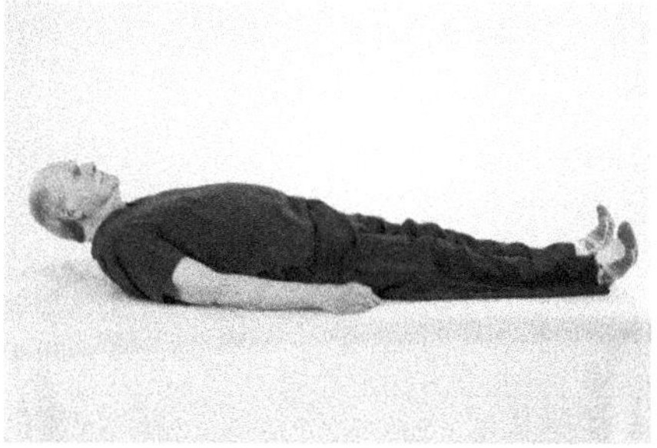

1. Lay on your back on the floor or other fairly firm surface.
2. Place your hands on your chest.
3. Roll your head and shoulders off the surface (figure 12-10a).
4. Hold that position until your abdominal muscles burn.
5. Slowly lower your head and shoulders back to the surface.
6. Repeat until your abdominal wall burns as soon as you roll your head and shoulders off the surface.
7. Repeat daily.

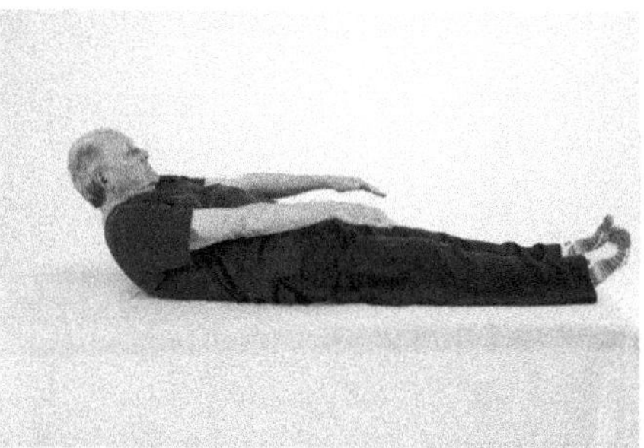

Once you have gotten this down well, change the exercise so that you lift your whole upper body off the surface, but do not sit all the way up (figure 12-10b). Once you start performing this version of the crunch add the second half of the exercise:

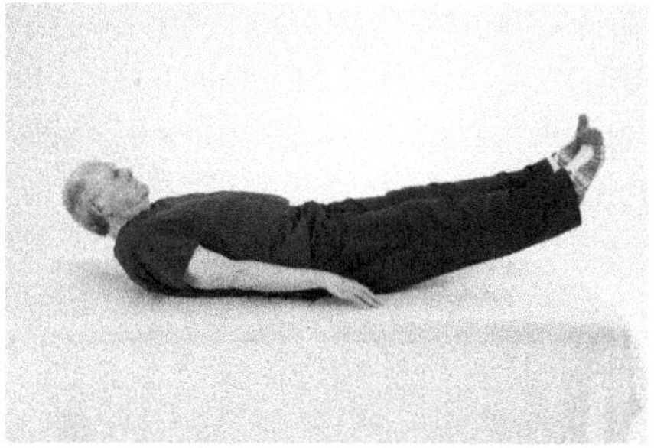

1. Continue to lie on your back on the floor or other fairly firm surface.
2. Place your hands on your chest.
3. Lift your feet and legs about six inches off the surface (figure 12-10c).
4. Hold that position until your abdominal muscles burn.
5. Slowly lower your legs and feet back to the surface.
6. Repeat until your abdominal wall burns as soon as you lift your legs and feet off the surface.

When you are able to hold your upper body off the surface for at least three minutes and your legs off the surface for three minutes as well, you are ready for the final version of this exercise.

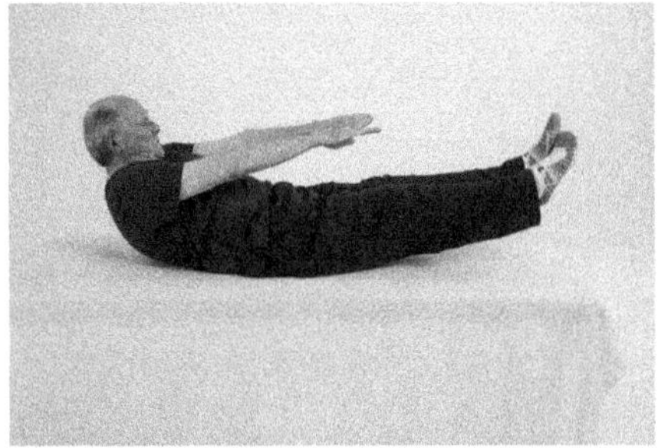

1. Lay on your back on the floor or other fairly firm surface.
2. Place your hands on your chest.
3. Simultaneously lift your upper body and legs and feet off the surface. This will put you in a shallow "V" (figure 12-10d).
4. Hold this position until your abdominal muscles begin to burn.
5. Lower your upper body and legs to the surface.
6. Repeat until your abdominal muscles begin to burn as soon as you get into the "V" position.

The final target is to be able to hold this "V" position for about five minutes. At this point you can simply repeat the five minute "V" crunch once a day. If you can do this, your abdominal muscles will certainly be able to carry their share of the load. This will take a load off your low back.

THE PLANK

Over the past couple of years, several studies have evaluated a range of exercises that are thought to have positive effects on developing and maintaining core strength. Surprisingly, the most effective is the Plank which comes to us from yoga. The version here is focused on developing and maintaining the core strength necessary to operate and protect the low back. It is not about developing washboard abs. It is simply incredibly effective in giving us core strength and endurance.

It can be performed either on the hands with outstretched arms like the pushup position or more comfortably with the elbows and forearms on the ground.

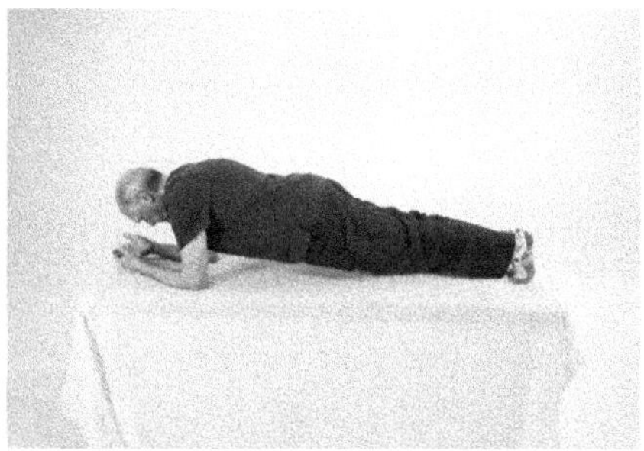

1. Start on your elbows or hands and knees.
2. Move your feet backward until your legs are straight and you are resting on your toes and forearms or hands.
3. Your body should be one straight line (figure 12-11). Do not look in front of you, but instead keep your head and neck in line with the rest of your spine and legs.
4. Hold this position as long as you can, then drop back to your knees.
5. That is the whole exercise. Repeat daily.

When you can hold the plank for two minutes without stopping you have reached your goal. Thereafter, simply do the Plank each day for two minutes. Your core muscles will now be sufficient to support your low back in most daily activity, even in the face of spinal arthritis, disc degeneration or even stenosis.

CHAPTER 13
Hips, Groin and Pelvis

Think of the pelvis as a bowl. It is oval in shape, longer side to side than front to back. It is largely made of three bones that are curved plates. This bowl is the platform that allows us to walk upright on two legs. Our legs attach to the outside of the bowl at the hip joints. The hip sockets are on the surface of the bowl and receive the ball of the femur. At the bottom of the bowl is a large opening closed by a combination of muscles, tendons and ligaments. Through that bottom opening come the anus, the urethra to allow our bladder to empty, and our sex organs. Inside the bowl we find three of the major organ systems of the body. These three organ systems in the abdomen include the digestive system, the urinary system, and the female reproductive organs and part of the male reproductive organs.

On the back side of the pelvis, the sacrum acts as the base on which the lumbar spine rests. The pelvis then plays a central role in not only our musculoskeletal system but also a significant interactive role with our visceral systems. Abnormal function in any of the elements of the pelvis can have major effects on posture and mobility, produce significant musculoskeletal pain, and even affect the operation of the visceral systems nestled within.

STRUCTURE OF THE PELVIS

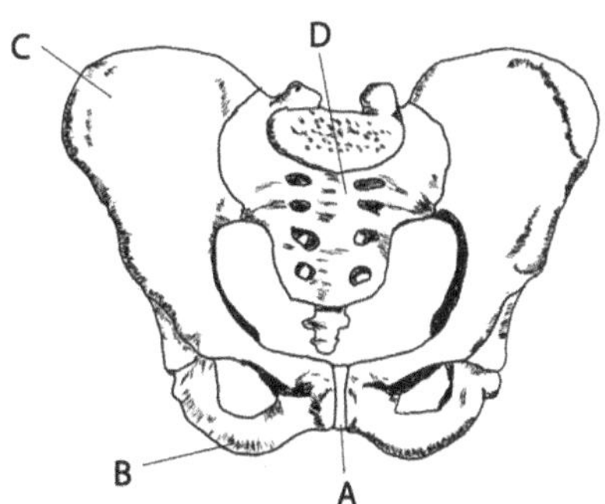

Two bones that make up the pelvis are called the *innominates* (fig. 13-1c). The third bone in the pelvis bowl is the sacrum. For the sake of simplicity, we will refer to the two innominate bones as the pelvic bones. In the embryo, each pelvic bone is the result of the fusion of several flat bones, the *ischium, acetabulum, pubes* and *ilium*. At the bottom of the pelvic bones are ring-shaped structures on which we sit, called the ischia or sitz bones (Figure 13-1b). Likewise, the sacrum develops from the fusion of five vertebrae. By the time of birth, the fusions are largely complete. Together the two pelvic bones form most of the bowl, narrowing to a bar in front, the pubis. The two pubic halves are joined to each other in front by cartilage (Fig. 13-1a). At the back side of the pelvis, each pelvic bone has a complex "L" shaped joint with the sacrum (Fig. 13-1d). The sacral joint is covered by very thick connective tissue front and back that suspends the sacrum between the two pelvic bones.

The pelvic bones and the sacrum, together with the hip and leg joints and the lumbar spine, form a complex movable structure. This structure allows us to stand upright, walk on two legs, carry objects, bend and stoop, and change from standing to sitting or squatting and back again. Limitation of motion in any one of these four elements will always compromise the overall ability to perform these normal human tasks. Such compromises inevitably are accompanied by pain.

THE PELVIC BONES

The pelvic bones are complex in shape. They also have quite a number of muscles that attach between them and the legs, low back and ribs. The muscles of the abdominal wall and low back attach to the pelvic bones, as do those that make up the pelvic floor. The buttocks and all of the thigh muscles attach to the pelvic bones as well. All of these muscles come into play as we stand, walk, or change position from sitting to standing or vice versa.

Pelvic dysfunctions have been discussed many times in previous chapters. In this book many of the patients discussed have had a problem that was termed an "up-slipped innominate" where the half pelvis on one side appears to be pushed superior, shortening the leg on that side. When standing, the upper lateral hip or the top of our pelvis will be higher and the shoulder on the same side will be lower. Inevitably this produces pain, although not always at the affected hip.

Although osteopathic literature has for many years suggested that the up-slipped innominate involved an upward shearing of half of the pelvis. In truth that is probably not possible. It is not uncommon for the leg length difference from an up-slipped innominate to be as much as ¾ inch when measured with the patient lying on his or her back. To actually generate that much difference by shearing the pelvic bone upward would totally destroy the joints between the sacrum and the pelvic bones. This joint is termed the sacroiliac joint. The joint is not destroyed in an up-slipped innominate. A more reasonable explanation would be that the pelvis is tilted at the sacroiliac joint so that the upper lateral rim is closer to the body midline and thus higher than that of the opposite side. In any case, one strategy to correct this problem has been to introduce a traction tug from the ankle.

The up-slipped innominate is not the only type of dysfunction that can affect the pelvic bones. Simply stumbling can rotate one pelvic bone forward and the other backward, also producing a difference in leg lengths. This makes it difficult for the average person to determine what has really occurred. When my patients visit elsewhere, they often will have someone gently tug on the short leg when they can't find an osteopathic physician to treat them.

THE SACRUM

Much of sacral dysfunction has traditionally been defined in terms of the interactions between the sacrum and its neighbors, the lumbar spine and the pelvic bones. The sacrum is a wedge-shaped bone between the two pelvic bones (Fig. 13-1d). The top of the sacrum is flat, like the bodies of the vertebrae. This makes a great deal of sense because the sacrum is created by fusing vertebrae after we are born. The lowest lumbar vertebra sits on top of the sacrum with all other vertebrae balanced above. The sacrum is suspended between the two pelvic bones by thick ligaments. As a result, the sacrum is one of the elements that moves when we move our bodies in walking, bending, stretching, sitting or lying down. Some MDs and, in particular, many orthopedic surgeons believe that there is no motion of the sacrum in relation to the two pelvic bones. We now have clear data showing the sacrum can move in relation to the pelvic bones, even if that movement is only 4 mm (roughly ¼ inch) in any particular direction.

As is the case between the vertebrae of the spine, nerves exit from the sacrum. Unlike the spine, the nerves exit to the front side of the sacrum where they join with the great sciatic nerve coming from the lumbar vertebrae. The sciatic nerve runs down in front of the sacrum before turning laterally towards the hip joint, exiting the pelvis below the lowest part of the sacroiliac joint.

Sometimes if there is enough vertical force, as when we take a hard fall, the sacrum will appear to be jammed down along the sacroiliac joints between the two halves of the pelvis. The normally mobile sacrum is now more or less immobilized. It is easy to understand how this can happen.

The sacrum is shaped like a wedge and the spine sits on top of it. When we fall, the parts of the pelvis that are termed the "sitz bones," hit and stop moving, but the upper body, spine and sacrum still have some momentum driven by gravity. The result is wedging the sacrum between the two halves of the bony pelvis like a keystone in an arch. When the sacrum is "jammed" we experience more back pain and stiffness or hip pain, because an element that is normally mobile has been frozen. Freeing the impacted sacrum provides significant relief. There are other events that can produce a similar jamming of the sacrum. One of the most common occurs when we plop onto a seat rather than letting ourselves down using our muscles (same mechanism as a fall but less force). Sometimes sneezing or coughing while sitting can cause the same problem. Sometimes lifting a heavy object inappropriately can produce a jammed sacrum.

PIRIFORMIS AND SCIATICA

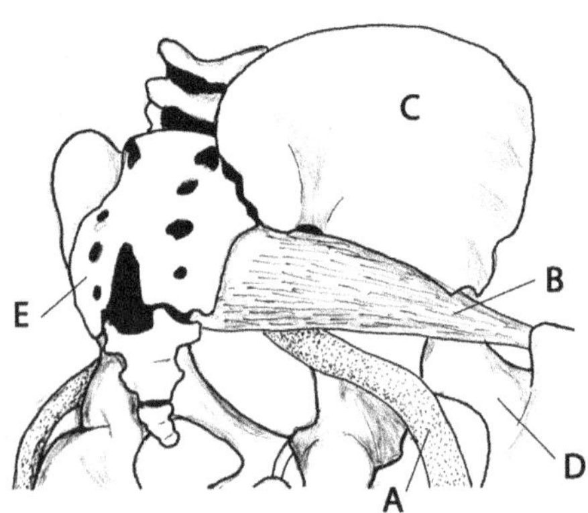

The piriformis muscle attaches to the front of the sacrum. The piriformis passes out from the inside of the pelvis, with its other end attaching to the femur. The femur is our thigh bone. The femur looks like a hockey stick with the upper head on a short horizontal shaft that bends at the greater trochanter (Fig. 13-2d) to become the long shaft we call the thigh bone (see also Fig. 17-3a). When we feel our "hip bone" we are pressing on that trochanter. The piriformis muscle tendon (Fig. 13-2b) attaches to the greater trochanter (Fig. 13-2d). The sciatic nerve (Fig. 13-2a) runs down the front face of the sacrum and then bends laterally to pass out of the pelvis along with the piriformis muscle.

THE GLUTEAL MUSCLES

The gluteal muscles are commonly referred to as the buttock or butt muscles. There are four primary muscles involved, the gluteus minimus, gluteus maximus, gluteus medius and piriformis. The first three have their origins on the dish shaped curve of the pelvic bone (Fig. 13-2c) and attach to the upper long bone of the leg, the femur. As noted above, the piriformis has its origin on the front of the sacrum (Fig. 13-2e), passes out from the inside of the pelvis along with the sciatic nerve, and also attaches to the upper femur.

THE PELVIS AND PAIN

Over the years the majority of my musculoskeletal patients have come to me because of pain. Frequently that pain has been in the low back, hip, groin, or leg. Most of the time they and the surgeons and pain management doctors who have tried to treat them have diagnosed the cause as being either the spine or the hip joint and treated them accordingly. When treatment for low back pain fails, typically the diagnosis shifts to the leg and treatment is adjusted accordingly. Often the patient has been to physical therapists, massage therapists or chiropractors who may have identified muscular or tendon elements of the pelvis and treated them. Sometimes the patient has found some diminishment of their pain for brief periods. However, in too many cases the relief they receive is at best inconsistent.

In too many cases, treatment failed because these other practitioners do not perform the kind of detailed diagnosis I use daily. What you don't look for you may not see. The patients often come to me as a last resort. Some of these patients have already had surgery, maybe even multiple surgeries. Again, the outcome of those surgeries has been no improvement in pain and perhaps even a worsening of their pain.

Remember the classical osteopathic understanding of such patients is based on a couple of interlocking ideas. First, the surgery itself does not leave the body in a normal anatomical and physiological state. As was discussed before, even the most skilled surgeon cannot completely restore tissue to its natural state. In many cases the surgeon intentionally had to change the structure by fusing some elements and introducing metal artificial parts to supplement or replace what was naturally present. Second, the initial problem itself may have had little to do with the operation. Even though spinal stenosis may have been the diagnosis from X-ray or CT scan or MRI, frequently there is little evidence that the stenosis was the actual cause of pain. The actual cause for the pain could have been muscle, tendon, ligament and joint structural imbalances in the pelvis caused by trauma or a gait disturbance. If the accumulated structural imbalances cannot be spontaneously corrected by the body, no amount of surgery will correct the problem. In fact, surgery, being a form of trauma, may make things worse.

I would like to be able to say that treating these patients with manual medicine is always successful in eliminating chronic low back and pelvis pain. Unfortunately, that is not always the case. Patients generally do get more relief from the kind of detailed neural, muscle and bone diagnosis and the related manipulative treatment than they did before seeing me. It may last for several weeks after each treatment, and subsequent treatments continue to be successful. However, some of the pain may return and the patient returns seeking repeat treatment. When I ask them about their satisfaction with their treatment, even though there is no permanent relief from their pain, the answers I get are typified by one of my older patients. She told me "Before I came to see you, I had continuous pain for seven years. Even in my sleep I had pain. In all that time, I had relief from the pain for no more than a day at most. Even the narcotics and shots didn't help. Now I have a couple days of complete relief after most of your treatments. After that the pain begins to come back slowly. Even those few days at a time are wonderful."

Because of their pain, most of these patients have stopped any form of exercise and stretching. Even the encouragement of the physical therapist has not been enough to overcome the psychological and physical block produced by pain. Therefore, most of these people have become both weak and stiff. Getting someone who has chronic pain back into an exercise and stretching regimen is not just a goal, but a necessity.

CHAPTER 14
Helping the Pelvis

Most of the exercises in this chapter have more to do with stretching and relaxing muscles and joints rather than strengthening the muscles. Actual strengthening exercises should be part of everyone's daily routine. Over the years I have found walking, swimming, aqua-aerobics, bicycling, dancing, Pilates, working out at a gym and the Oriental routines of the martial arts, Tai Chi, and movement-based yoga all benefit us greatly. My advice has always been to find some form of exercise that you can enjoy and do it at least three or four times a week. I have found that as people age there is a tendency to move away from the more vigorous forms of exercise. Therefore, I tend to emphasize those that seniors seem more willing to incorporate in their lives like walking, swimming, aquatic exercise, Tai Chi and yoga. All are good for general stretching, strength and coordination and all except swimming also help with the balance issues that become more common with age.

The exercises that follow in this chapter are more specifically aimed at helping stretch muscles, tendons and joint capsules around the pelvis and thigh. When these become too tight, they can severely limit our ability to walk any distance and can cause a lot of pain in legs, hips and the lower back.

SUPINE KNEE TO CHEST

This exercise is very useful to relieve tension in the low back, pelvic floor and hamstring muscles. It is performed in bed, on the floor or on a mat.

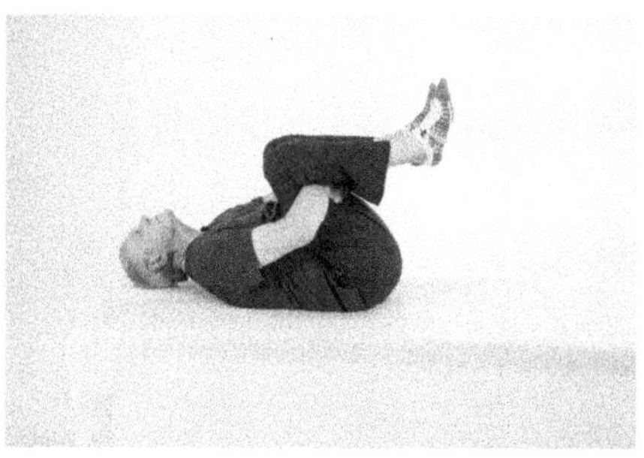

1. Lie on your back. Bend your knees.
2. Bring both of your knees as close to your chest as you can (Fig.14-1). If there are problems with the low back and hips, you might only get to 90 degrees or about the position of sitting on a chair.
3. Grasp the top of the lower legs just below the knees with your hands. If your arms are not long enough, grasp the ends of a rolled towel or a strap with each hand and wrap it around the front of your knees.
4. Without letting your legs win, gently push your knees away from your chest as if you were trying to straighten them out. Do this in three brief pulses.
5. Use your hands to pull your knees a little closer to your chest and hold this new position for about ten seconds. Repeat three times before allowing your legs to lay flat on the floor or bed.

GLUTEUS MUSCLE STRETCH

Three of the buttock or hip muscles on each side oppose each other in their actions when the hips are flexed at 90 degrees. Gluteus maximus, the biggest of the muscles, will pull the leg to the side (termed abduction) when the hip is flexed. The other two muscles, gluteus medius and minimus, will tend to pull the leg toward the opposite side of the body (adduction) when the hip is flexed. When these muscles are tight you may feel tension, tenderness or pain in the middle of your buttock. Therefore, to stretch these hip muscles will require two separate moves.

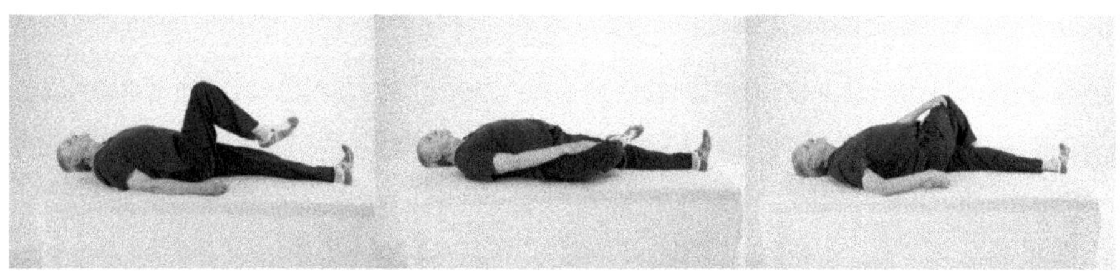

1. Lie on your back.
2. Bend the knee and the hip so that the hip is at 90 degrees (Fig. 14-2a).
3. Bring the knee out to the side and place your hand on the inside of the thigh or knee (Fig. 14-2b).

4. Gently but briefly push your leg up against the restraining hand but do not push strongly enough for the leg to win. Do this three times. Then release the restraining hand.

6. Now move your leg so the knee is up toward the ceiling or even better across your midline toward the opposite side.

7. Place one or both restraining hands against the outside of that thigh or knee (Fig. 14-2c).

8. Gently but briefly push the leg against the restraining hand(s) three times.

9. Relax and let your leg straighten out.

GLUTEUS MUSCLE RELAXATION

Voluntarily relaxing a muscle can be as effective a treatment as stretching. To relax gluteus maximus lie on your back. Bend the knee and the hip on the side to be relaxed at right angles. Now bring the knee to the side close to the surface you are lying on. In this position, gluteus maximus will be relaxed. Hold this position for 2 to 3 minutes and then restore the leg to a stretched-out position. Gluteus maximus should remain relaxed.

PIRIFORMIS STRETCH

Piriformis is a buttock muscle that is notorious for its effects when it is tight or in spasm. It is one of the few muscles that has an attachment directly to the sacrum. It comes out from in front of the sacrum through the sciatic notch. It then attaches to the outside of the hip. The sciatic notch is called that because the sciatic nerve comes out in parallel with the piriformis muscle (see Chapter 13). Sometimes when piriformis is in spasm it actually pinches or compresses the sciatic nerve. This can cause pain, tingling, or numbness that radiates down the leg past the knee to the foot. This is one cause of sciatica.

To stretch the piriformis muscle yourself you can use either a seated or a lying position. Let us start with the lying down position.

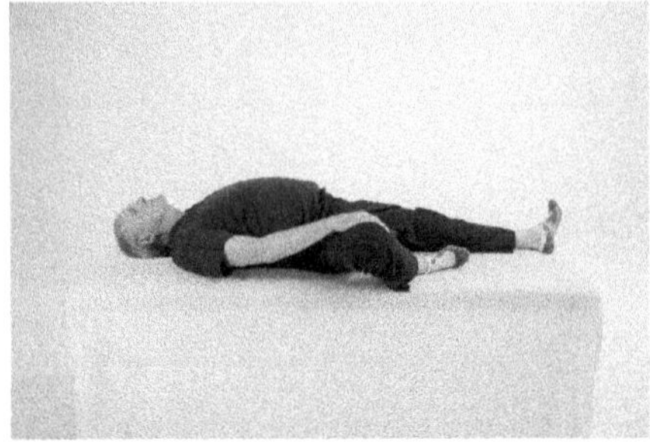

1. Bend the knee and hip on the affected side and place the ankle and foot near your other thigh.
2. Let the knee relax towards the floor.
3. Place your hand on the inside of the knee (Fig. 14-3a).
4. Gently push the knee upward against the hand but don't let the knee win.
5. Repeat three times and then allow the knee to further relax. It will fall further towards the floor and the piriformis will relax.

Sometimes the piriformis won't relax enough, and in this case, you will need to do the following step:

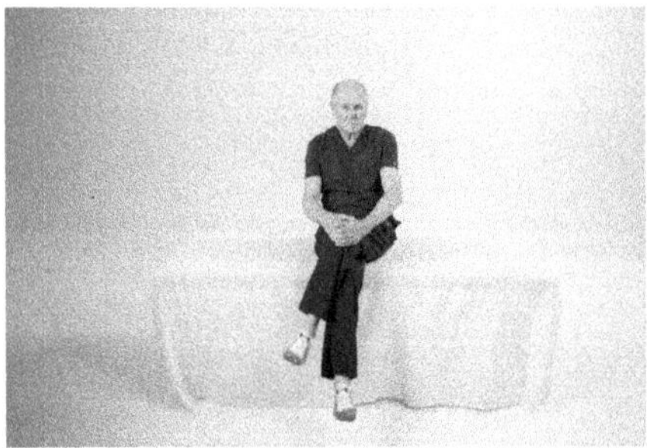

1. In a seated position cross your legs so that the foot of the affected piriformis is outside the other thigh.
2. Place your hand against the outside of the knee of the affected leg (Fig. 14-3c).
3. Gently use the affected leg to press laterally against your hand, and repeat three times.
4. Relax and use your hand to press the knee of the affected leg further to the opposite side.

You can perform the same type of piriformis relaxation seated. Sometimes this stretch is more effective than the lying down stretch.

PIRIFORMIS RELAXATION

To relax piriformis the positioning is the same as the stretch. To determine which of the two positions will be most effective at relaxing the muscle try each one. One of them will provide palpable relaxation. That is the position you will hold for at least two minutes.

PSOAS STRETCH

The psoas is an unusual muscle that starts on the lateral parts of the low back but runs down through the pelvis to attach to the femur. Activating psoas causes the upper leg to flex at the hip. When you bend over at the hips or lift your thigh or leg that is the psoas. If it is tight on both sides, you will stand and walk bent over at the hips. If it is tight on just one side, you won't be able to straighten up fully on that side. Trying to straighten up and stand erect with tight psoas causes pain from your low back into your groin. There are two stretches that can help with a tight psoas muscle. The first is done lying on your back at the edge of the bed.

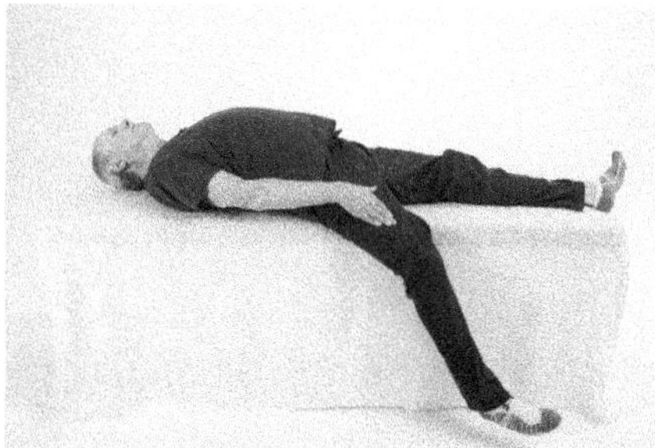

1. The tight psoas side should be at the edge of the bed.
2. Drop that leg off the side of the bed, placing your hand on that thigh (Fig. 14-4a).
3. Gently lift the thigh against the resistance from your hand. Repeat three times.
4. Let the leg drop towards the floor.

The second psoas stretch is a little more complicated. For those with yoga experience you might recognize the similarities with part of the warrior pose. I actually first learned this as a teenager taking judo.

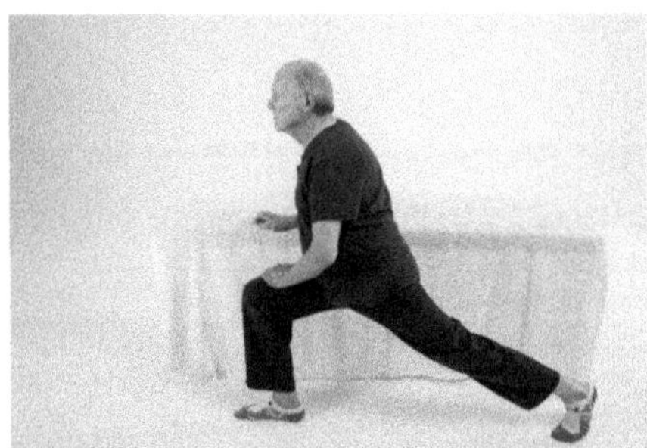

1. Stand next to a sturdy object like a table or desk if you have problems with your balance.
2. The leg with the tight psoas will be behind your pelvis.
3. Go into a lunge with the other leg flexed at the hip and knee. Keep the leg with the tight psoas straight at the knee but stretched backward as far as possible at the hip (Fig. 14-4b).
4. Go as far into the lunge as the tight psoas allows.
5. By holding that position, try to activate tight psoas by briefly trying to swing the back leg forward. It should not move but the muscle will be isometrically activated. Repeat three times.
6. After the third activation, relax into a deeper lunge.

QUADRICEPS STRETCH

The quadriceps muscle is the big muscle on the front of the thigh. It actually consists of four strap muscles that attach to the pelvis and to the knee cap. If the knee is bent, the quadriceps will pull on the knee and straighten the knee out. When the quadriceps muscles are tight it is very difficult to bend the knee. Sometimes they can keep the knee from bending even as much as 90 degrees. The knee should be able to bend about 165 degrees, so that the calf touches the back of the thigh.

The stretching exercise for quadriceps can be performed either standing or lying on the other side. If you are performing this stretch standing, I recommend having a stable chair or table next to you that you can hold onto with the opposite hand.

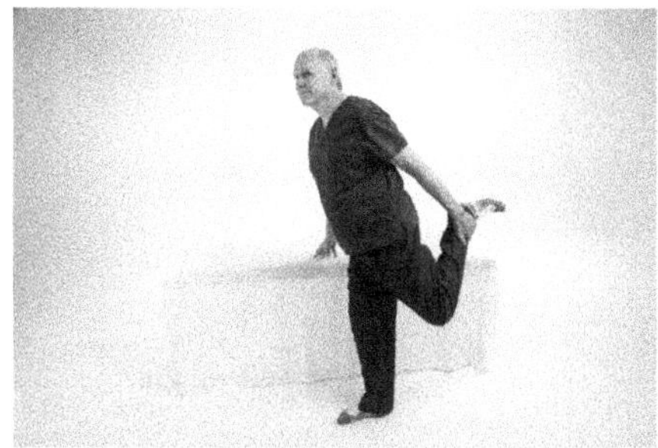

1. Bend your knee so that you can grab the ankle with your hand. If you cannot bend your knee enough to grab it with your hand, use a belt or a strap around that ankle and grab the strap with your hand.
2. Pull your ankle up toward your buttock with your hand until you feel tension in the front of the thigh (Fig. 14-5).
3. Gently and briefly try to straighten the knee out against the resistance from your hand. Do not use so much force that the leg wins.
4. Repeat three times.
5. Now gently pull the ankle up towards the buttock with your hand.

HAMSTRINGS STRETCH ONE LEG

The hamstrings are the muscles on the back of the thigh. There are four muscles altogether that make up the hamstrings. They attach to the bony prominence (ischium) below the buttock and on the backside of the knee. Their job is to bend the knee and to help extend the thigh backwards at the hip.

Many of us have very tight hamstrings. Sometimes this is because the form of exercise we do automatically tightens the hamstrings. Most of us do not routinely perform stretches for the hamstrings. If the hamstrings are too tight, it is difficult to bend forward at the waist. If the hamstrings are tighter on one side than the other, they may cause an imbalance in the pelvis. This can affect walking, sitting, stair climbing and any other activity that requires flexing the thigh. Tight hamstrings can also contribute significantly to low back pain.

There are several ways to stretch the hamstrings of one leg at a time. The easiest is performed lying on your back.

1. Try to bring the affected knee to your chest.
2. Wrap your hands around the thigh just above the knee (Fig. 14-6a).
3. Gently press the leg away from your chest, but do not allow the leg to win.

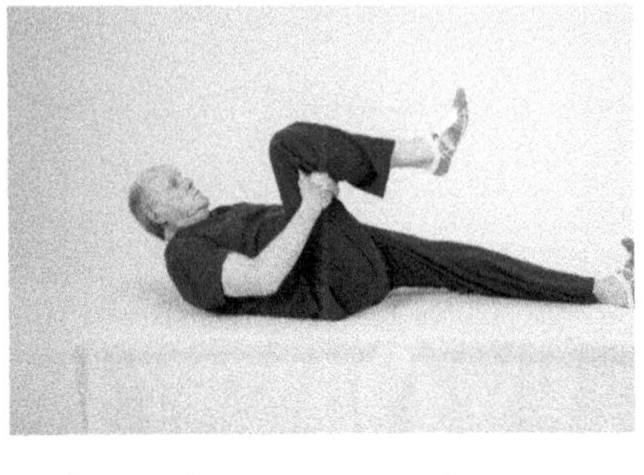

4. After three quick presses, pull the knee closer to your chest.

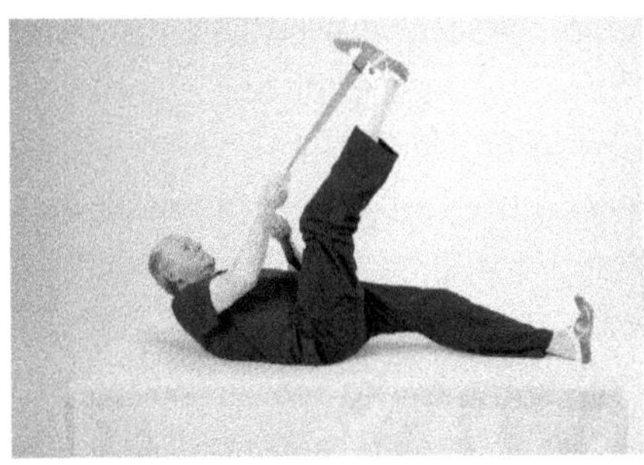

A variation on this is commonly taught but harder to do. This uses a strap around the ankle or foot and pulls the mostly straight leg towards the chest (Fig 14-6b). This is considerably more advanced and is not advised unless the hamstrings are pretty loose already.

Another hamstring stretch, commonly called the runners stretch, is performed standing. In the standard runners stretch, the leg that is being stretched is placed upon an elevated surface like the seat of the chair. The person then bends the torso forward and tries to grab the foot. Not only is this not successful in many cases, but it has the possibility of tearing the hamstrings if it is performed too forcefully. A much safer variation is as follows.

1. Stand erect. Place the heel of the leg to be stretched on an elevated surface.
2. Gently bend forward along the leg until you feel tension begin to develop at the back of the thigh.

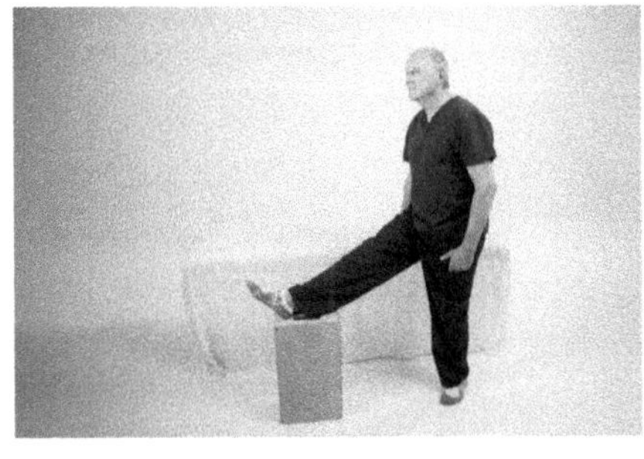

3. Holding that position, wrap your hands around the knee, the calf or the foot wherever your stretch reaches (Fig. 14-6c).
4. Now gently, but briefly, try to straighten up. Repeat three times.
5. You will find that if you bend your body further forward you will be able to bend further before tension reoccurs in the back of your thigh.

HAMSTRINGS STRETCH BOTH LEGS

There is a simple standing stretch for the hamstrings that I use daily. It is also quite effective.

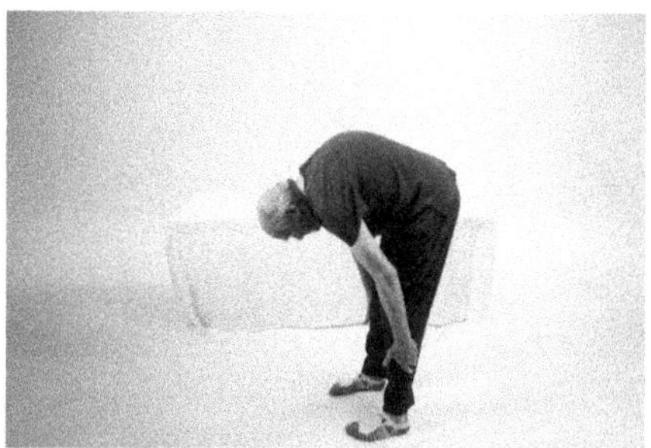

1. In a standing position bend forward. The bending should be at the hips rather than the low back.
2. When you reach a position where there is tension at the back of both thighs, reach down with your hands and grasp the leg (Fig. 14-6d). In some cases, you may have to start with grabbing above the knee. This is not a problem. If you can grab your feet from this position, you do not have tight hamstrings.
3. Gently try to straighten up to an erect position. Once again you will prevent that by holding on to your legs with your hands. Perform three brief straightening attempts.
4. Now, as you relax from the last attempt to straighten you will find that your hands are able to reach further down on your legs.

HIP ADDUCTORS STRETCH

The adductors are the muscles on the inside of your thigh. There are four of them altogether. As a group their job is to move your legs together. When you try to squeeze something with your legs you are using the hip adductors. Most of the time, tightness in the hip adductors is signaled by pain along the middle side of the knee and difficulties spreading the legs.

To stretch the hip adductor muscles, stand facing a stable chair back or table. You will want to have your hands on that object for balance and to help you return to a normal standing position after you have done the stretch.

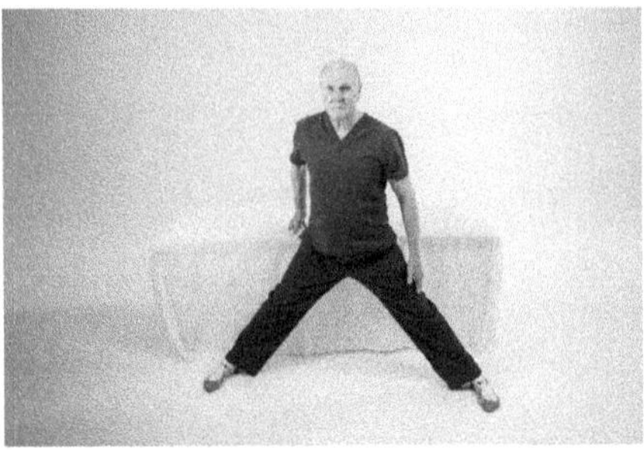

1. Move your feet apart as far as you can comfortably. You should feel some tension along your inner thighs, but no pain (Fig. 14-7).
2. Keeping your feet in this position, try to bring your thighs together. As in previous stretches this should be brief and repeated three times.
3. Now try to spread your legs further apart by walking your feet out to the side.

STRENGTHENING HIP ADDUCTORS

For many of us, the inner thigh muscles are relatively weak. Stretching will help, but we also need to strengthen the muscles. The simplest method of doing so involves placing a fairly large ball between your knees and squeezing multiple times each day.

ILIOTIBIAL BAND STRETCH

The iliotibial band (IT band) is one of the thickest bands of connective tissue in the body. At the upper end of the iliotibial band is a muscle named the tensor fascia lata. Together with the gluteal muscles, the tensor fascia lata pulls on the iliotibial band to spread the legs apart. Together the iliotibial band and tensor fascia lata also stabilize the hip when standing. When one IT band is tight, we cannot move the leg towards the other side of the body. When it is tight, the tensor fascia lata and iliotibial band can cause significant pain over the lateral hip as well as the outer side of the thigh and knee.

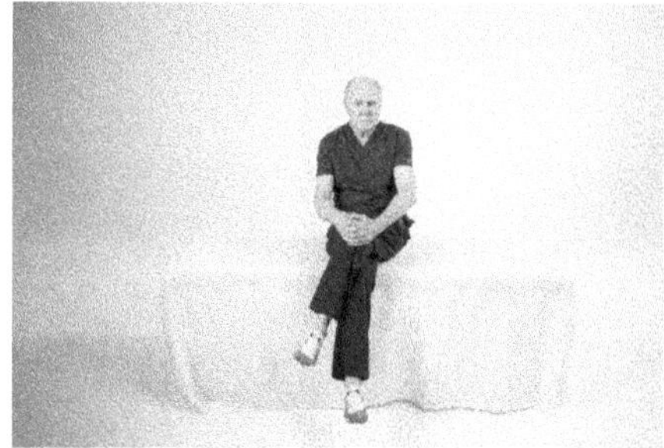

1. To stretch the iliotibial band and tensor fascia lata, cross your legs so that the leg of the affected side is on top of the other thigh.
2. Place your hand against the outside of the knee of the affected leg (Fig. 14-8).
3. Gently use the affected leg to press laterally against your hand and the outside of the other leg.
4. Repeat three times.
5. Relax and use your hand to press the knee of the affected leg further to the opposite side.

ILIOTIBIAL BAND RELAXATION

The easiest way to relax the iliotibial band and tensor fascia lata is to lie on your back. Bring the affected leg out to the side as far as you can easily. Simply lay there in this position for at least two minutes. There should be little tenderness in either the iliotibial band or tensor fascia lata after you have done this.

SELF-TREATMENTS FOR A PELVIS UP-SLIP

Sometimes we know when we have done something to cause the kind of pelvis imbalance that has been referred to throughout this book as an up-slipped pelvis or innominate. We step into a hole in the otherwise level grass and jar that leg and half of the pelvis. Similar jarring can be the result of stepping off a curb or missing a step. We may not feel any immediate pain, but treating the problem right after it occurs can prevent a whole lot of trouble.

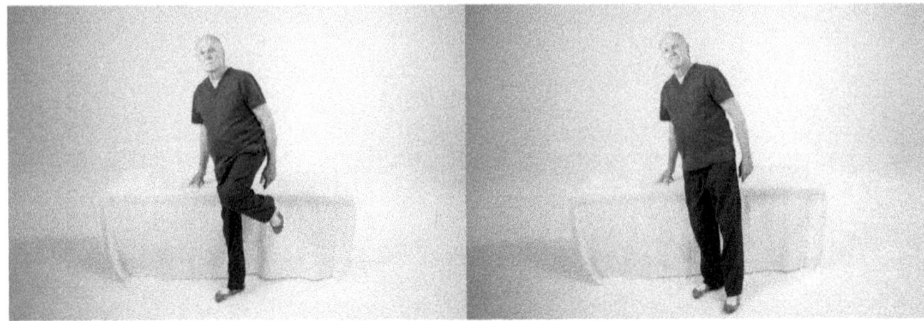

1. Lean against a stable object like a wall or signpost so that your weight is off the jarred leg and hip.
2. Partially flex the jarred knee and hip (Fig 14-9a).
3. Straighten the jarred leg with a thrust toward the ground (Fig. 14-9b).

At other times you may not be aware of what caused the pelvis to be so mis-aligned that one leg is short. The only clue is that you develop mild pain and discomfort in one of the buttocks. If you lie on your back on the floor, bed, or massage table you might be able to feel that one leg is shorter than the other. If you suspect you might have an up-slipped pelvis, have someone look at the ankles of your outstretched legs while you are lying on your back. Your legs should be stretched out, flat on the surface and parallel to each other. If one middle ankle bone (malleolus) is apparently closer to your pelvis than the other, that leg is functionally shortened and needs to be treated. To treat yourself lie on a bed or similar elevated surface:

1. Roll on your side with the short leg up in the air.
2. Move so that your pelvis is at the edge of the surface and your legs can dangle over the edge.
3. Holding your legs straight and together, let them sink below the level of the surface on which you are lying (Fig. 14-9c).
4. Continuing to hold them together, lift them so that they are at the level of the surface you are lying on.
5. Repeat three times.
6. After doing this you can recheck. Your legs should be the same length.

If all else fails, seek the help of an osteopathic physician or other musculoskeletal practitioner who knows how to diagnose and treat an up-slipped innominate.

SELF-TREATMENT FOR A JAMMED SACRUM

Recall that a jammed sacrum occurs when the sacrum and spine move inferior, but the rest of the pelvis has stopped moving. Typically, a person with a jammed sacrum will feel dull pressure, stiffness and pain across the low back below the tops of the pelvis.

The primary self-treatment for a jammed sacrum may be a bit difficult for some people to perform. It is quite effective whether the jamming occurred recently or at some point in the past.

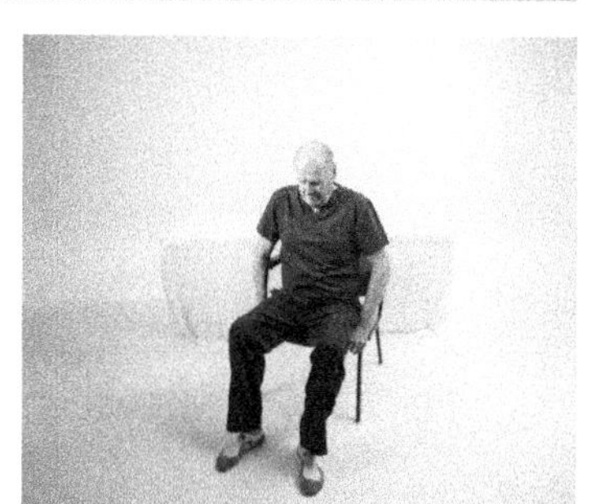

1. Sit on a chair with your feet on the floor. Leave enough space between your calves and the chair to allow your forearms to fit under your thighs.
2. Sitting upright, stabilize your shoulders by placing your elbows on the arms of the chair or hands on the seat of the chair.
3. Slowly tilt your head and neck backwards (Fig. 14-10a) and then forwards (Fig. 14-10b). As your head and neck move forward, they will lift the whole spine and sacrum. (Do this three times.)
4. Lean forward so your abdomen and chest are on your thighs.
5. Wrap your arms around your thighs and grasp your forearms with your hands (Fig. 14-10c).
6. Attempt to lift your torso off of your thighs. This is not a contest, so lift gently. The idea is to isometrically activate your back muscles, particularly in the lower back.

7. After the third torso lift unclasp your forearms. Move your hands to the tops of your thighs.
8. Push yourself into an erect sitting position with your arms (Fig. 14-10d). Do not straighten up using your back muscles. This completes the self-release exercise.

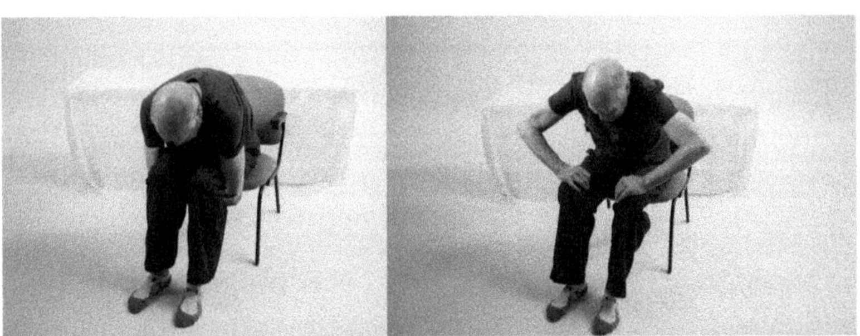

Another treatment for the jammed sacrum that is more likely to work when the problem arose within the past day or two is somewhat easier to perform.

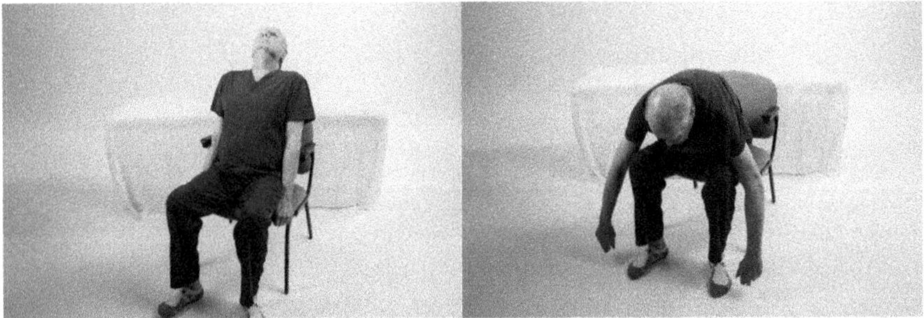

1. Sit on a stable surface with room to lean back. Place your hands behind you on the surface.
2. Lean back, supporting yourself on your hands (Fig. 14-11a). Do this for 20 seconds.
3. Now slowly bend forward starting with your head and working down to the low back (Fig. 14-11b).
4. Move your arms forward.
5. Now push yourself back into an upright position with your arms. Do not use your back muscles.

A third treatment for a sacrum that is jammed can be done if the second one does not work:

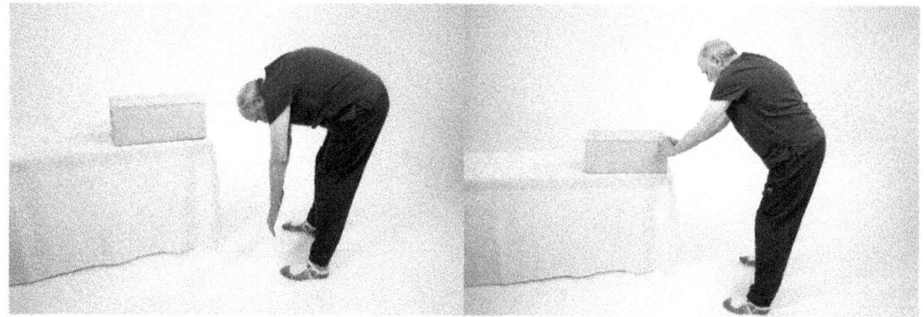

1. Stand in front of a cabinet corner with your feet spread apart, wider than your shoulders. You should be an arm's length from the cabinet.

2. Bend forward toward the cabinet as far as you can with your hands approaching the floor (Fig. 14-12a). If you can actually touch the floor, don't.

3. Hold this position for 20 seconds.

4. Use your hands on the cabinet edge to push yourself back upright (Fig. 14-12b). Do not use your back muscles to straighten to an upright position.

5. Once erect, keep your feet spread apart and thrust your pelvis forward one time. Then return to a normal upright position.

6. Bring your feet together. This completes the exercise.

CHAPTER 15
The Neck

There are seven bones in the cervical spine. With the exception of the top two cervical vertebrae, each neck bone (cervical vertebra) consists of a part like a hockey puck, the vertebral body. Between each vertebral body and those above and below are the discs. The disc is a gel-filled fibrous body that is flexible, as if it were made of rubber. This allows one vertebra to bend forward and backward and sideways on the vertebra below it. Behind the vertebral body is a boney ring that surrounds and protects the spinal cord. In order to keep the vertebrae from moving too far relative to each other, there are bony projections aligned vertically off the ring. As in the rest of the spine these are termed facet joints. Each cervical vertebra has eight of these bony projections, four pointed up and four pointed down. The projections pointed up are oriented to slide against those pointed down on the vertebra above. Because of how these joints are aligned, movements on the diagonal are more likely to cause joint binding and result in motion restriction and pain in the neck.

SPINAL ARTHRITIS, DISC DEGENERATION AND CERVICAL SPINAL STENOSIS

Arthritis can develop in the cervical spine just as it does in the rest of the spine. In most cases, arthritis of the cervical spine is a result of osteoarthritis. Spinal arthritis is associated with decreased range of motion that develops over time, stiffness and sometimes pain. It may involve some grating sound, as if there was sand in the neck. On X-rays we see bone spurs between the bodies of the vertebrae and/or from the facet joints. In most cases we also see a decrease in some of the space between the bodies of the neck vertebrae. This means that the discs are degenerating or collapsing. Similar findings are seen on CT scans or an MRI of the neck. Most of the time these signs of an arthritic neck worsen as we get older, but they may be seen under the age of 50 after an accident or trauma to the neck. By itself, cervical osteoarthritis rarely causes pain. However, it can contribute to pain by forcing the neck muscles to work harder and more of the time than normal. In other cases where arthritis limits the range of motion, neck muscle atrophy can develop with its attendant pain. Finally, neck pain in the presence of arthritis may occur when there is an additional injury, strain, or other event that produces an imbalance in the range of motion of at least a couple of the neck vertebrae. Osteoarthritis of the neck also seems to contribute to poor spontaneous recovery from the pain-producing event.

If there is a significant narrowing of the nerve outlet due to a combination of arthritic spurs, disc bulges and soft tissue overgrowth, it is termed stenosis. If the stenosis or narrowing is at a nerve outlet it can lead to a pinched nerve and pain. Similarly, if there is stenosis in the central canal where the spinal cord is found it can pinch the spinal cord, often causing significant pain that may not be confined to the neck or upper body. Most of the time stenosis, like spinal arthritis, does not produce much pain, although it, too, can contribute to significant reduction in the normal range of motion of the neck.

Mostly, pain in the arthritic neck is due to the strain a restriction puts on the muscles and tendons that move the neck. Since these are also guarding against any motion that will trigger further pain, we end up with another vicious pain cycle. Not using the neck muscles causes weakening and, in extreme cases, muscle atrophy. Once the neck muscles weaken or atrophy, trying to move the neck causes pain. In turn, the pain is enough to keep us from attempting to turn the neck.

One patient came to see me more than 20 years ago with a complaint of pain in his neck. He was having difficulty with driving his car because he had to turn his body to see what was occurring on either side of his car. When I asked him to turn his head to the right, he was able to move it about 5 degrees (the normal range is about 70 degrees to each side). His movement to the left was imperceptible, in spite of his best efforts. When I tried to move his neck, even with my best manipulative method, I found I could only add about five degrees to his movement in either direction. Subsequent X-rays demonstrated significant disc degeneration and arthritis spurring.

At the second office visit, he felt his neck was less stiff and on evaluation he had preserved most of the range of motion he had left the office with after his first treatment. In addition to performing osteopathic manipulation on his neck (and the rest of his spine), I prescribed a series of neck exercises that I had found in an old osteopathic book from the early 1900s, the Four Quadrant Exercises (see Chapter 16).

Following my instructions, the patient admitted he could initially only do one or two of each movement. Over time he slowly built up to doing the full series daily. After six months of osteopathic manipulations every three or four weeks and the patient performing the neck exercises daily, he regained approximately 90 percent of normal range of motion in his neck. Years later he continued to do the neck exercises daily and enjoy virtually normal neck range of motion with minimal pain, stiffness or even discomfort even though there was no improvement in the arthritis and disc degeneration in his neck.

HERNIATED DISC

As in the rest of the spine, a cervical spinal disc can develop tears in its outer fiber ring. This allows the inner gel, or nucleus, of the disc to push out. Generally, this disc herniation happens on the back side of the disk, pushing into the spinal canal where the spinal cord and nerve roots are located. The disc wall tear and pushing out of the inner gel typically occurs when an unusual amount of force compresses the disc. Most often a cervical disc herniation occurs with the head and neck extended backward.

In such injuries there can be a fair amount of pain immediately. Probably little of the pain is produced by the actual tear. However, the soft tissues of the neck, including the muscles and connective tissues, are typically overstretched. Sometimes this strain is termed a "whiplash" injury. However, disc herniation can cause the disc material to press on the spinal cord or the spinal nerves as they leave the cervical spine. When the herniated disc presses on the spinal cord it may affect the whole body below the neck, and may affect both sensation (numbness, tingling and pain) and the ability to move our muscles (weakness and paralysis).

When the cervical nerves are compressed by a disc herniation, the compression will typically involve one side of the body, not both. With nerve compression you may see muscle weakness, pain and changes in sensation. The pattern of pain produced by a herniated disc tends to predict where the disc has herniated. When the lower cervical spine (C5 through C8) is involved, there may be pain, numbness and tingling down the arm beginning at the shoulder. For instance, a C6 nerve compression in the right cervical spine will produce abnormal sensations in the right thumb only. A C8 disc herniation will produce abnormal sensations in the ring and little fingers. The pain from a disc herniation can be somewhat more diffuse since the pain neurons (nociceptors) may spread up and down the spinal cord by a couple of levels before they terminate. Because of this the numbness and tingling are a better predictor of the level of the herniation than the neck pain.

A herniated cervical disc may not require surgery. The herniation often leaves some room for the nerve or spinal cord. Even if there is some evidence of sensory or muscle involvement from the herniation it can go away over time. About 90 percent of all disc herniations resolve symptomatically over four to six weeks. Most spine surgeons will give a course of oral steroids and allow some time to lapse before considering surgery. The steroid will lessen any swelling in the tissues around the nerve or spinal cord. Over time the disc material may well absorb back into the disc. The only indication for immediate surgery is if the herniation is causing paralysis or if the herniated disc material breaks free and therefore has no chance of being absorbed back into the disc.

BRACHIAL PLEXUS COMPRESSION

I have had many patients come to me with an MRI showing a right cervical disc herniation and numbness, tingling and pain in the right arm. I have also had many patients come to see me with sensory abnormalities and pain on the opposite side of the herniated disc. In most cases, the patient has already seen a spine surgeon. The surgeon did not think that the patient would benefit from surgery, leaving the patient confused because they do have a herniated disc, and in their mind that equates with surgery.

In a disc herniation, we need to give things time in order for the body to heal itself. In many cases pain, numbness and tingling down an arm may have little to do with the herniated disc. The most obvious case is when the disc herniation is above the level for the nerves to the arm (C2 through C4). It should be equally obvious that a disc herniation on one side of the spine cannot cause pain, numbness and tingling down the opposite arm since the spinal nerves only go to the body on the side of their origin.

How can we account for the discrepancy between the location of the disc herniation and the arm pain, numbness and tingling? Like the issue of sciatica and the lumbar spine, the nerves for the arm are frequently compressed outside the cervical spine.

As soon as the cervical nerves to the arm leave the spine, they gather together in bundles that together are termed the brachial plexus. These nerve bundles gather above the top of the first rib, passing between muscles that are termed the scalenes. The nerve bundles then run under the collar bone in the direction of the front of the shoulder. At the shoulder they pass over the anterior lateral chest wall and serratus anterior muscles but under the two pectoral muscles (the flat muscles on the front of the chest termed pectoralis major and pectoralis minor) before passing into the arm. In the upper arm the nerves run in a groove between the bicep and triceps muscles. They then pass the middle side of the elbow and into the forearm, across the wrist and into the palm of the hand in the groove called the carpal tunnel.

All along the path of the brachial plexus there are potential pinch points where the nerves can be compressed. At the base of the neck the first rib can be immobilized (remember all ribs move during breathing and as we move our spine). If the first rib is immobile, the scalene muscles are typically tight and can compress the brachial plexus. Fracture of the collar bone can compress these nerves. Pectoral muscle tightness or bursitis at the front of the shoulder can also compress the nerve. Tightness of the muscles and tendons at the elbow can compress these nerves. And last but not least, swelling or thickening of the tissues at the carpal tunnel can compress these nerves as they enter the hand.

Consider the case of one of my patients who presented with pain in his neck with some pain, numbness and tingling in his right arm. He was in his early 50s. He used to be quite active physically, but more recently had been spending much of his working day in front of a computer. He did, however, go to the gym once a week and enjoyed his golf outings on the weekend. He was stopped at a red light when his car was hit from behind by another car that failed to stop. His right hand was on the steering wheel. His seatbelt prevented any obvious injury. Even so, he developed an immediate pain in his neck. He was taken by ambulance to the local hospital. In the ER examination, a neck X-ray revealed only a flattening of the typical curve of the neck indicating a soft tissue injury or whiplash. He was sent home with orders to follow-up with his internist.

Within two days of his accident, he had developed pretty significant pain in his neck. More troubling was a pain down his right arm, with numbness and tingling into his hand. He felt his grip was weak even though he was right-handed. His internist sent him for an MRI of his cervical spine. When that revealed a disc herniation at C6 he was referred to a neurosurgeon who specializes in spinal surgery. The surgeon, however, did not advise surgery and instead put him on prednisone (a steroid) and sent him for physical therapy. Three weeks later the patient's neck pain was somewhat better but he still had pain, numbness, tingling and weakness in his right hand. He was referred to me by one of his golfing buddies.

When I first saw this patient, the first and most obvious fact was that his cervical disc herniation was fairly mild and was on the left, pushing on the left C6 nerve outlet. Clearly the neurosurgeon had made the right choice since the symptoms were on the right. I found that virtually his whole hand and arm were numb, and a simple light touch to his hand and wrist produced tingling. This pattern was not consistent with compression of a single nerve root at the spine. That, in turn, suggested that the problem might well be coming from a compression of the brachial plexus outside the spine.

As I evaluated the patient's neck and arm, I noted that his right first rib was clearly immobile and his scalene muscles were tight. He had a gap in the AC joint (acromial-clavicular) of the right shoulder which lies just above the brachial plexus and often produces pain and restriction in the shoulder. There was mild tenderness over both the middle and outside of the elbow, indicating that the muscles from the wrist and hand that attach there had been strained. And finally, there were restrictions in the bones that make up the base of the hand, restrictions that pushed on the carpal tunnel. This pattern is what is often called a multiple crush injury and could cause compression of the brachial plexus all along its course.

As I treated each site of potential compression along the course of his right brachial plexus, his numbness and tingling began to resolve. By the end of our first office visit his feeling of weakness, numbness and pain in his right arm had disappeared. At the follow-up office visit two weeks later he reported that he had had a couple of episodes of numbness and tingling in bed at night when he tried to rest his head on his hands while lying on his back. Otherwise, his only complaint was some pain in his neck and shoulders. Again, I treated his neck and the rest of his spine with osteopathic manipulative treatment. Since he also showed some signs of a right rib strain pattern that could affect the shoulder, I also treated that. I encouraged him to restart his exercise program. At a follow-up two weeks later, most of his problems had been resolved. He was worried about the herniated disc in his neck and that it might cause him problems in the future. I reassured him that it had not played a significant role in the symptoms from his accident and so probably would not mean much in the future. Most likely it would simply heal on its own. If he did develop similar symptoms in his left arm and thumb in the near future it could mean the disc had gotten worse.

If this patient's symptoms had developed initially on the same side as the disc herniation it would have made it a little harder to determine whether his problem was coming from the disc herniation. Most likely the surgeon would have pursued the same course and waited about a month before suggesting the next step. Most spine surgeons prefer to have a nerve conduction study performed to see if it can be determined where the nerves are being compressed. They might also suggest a trial of epidural injections in which a steroid is injected inside the spinal canal but outside the dura (a thick fascial tube that surrounds the spinal cord). These epidural injections often will calm inflammation enough that the symptoms resolve.

If such a patient comes to me before surgery, I typically suggest a short course of manipulation to determine whether the symptoms are totally or partly the result of compression along the course of the nerve outside the spine. If the symptoms resolve, then the problem was a brachial plexus compression rather than from the disc herniation.

CHAPTER 16
Helping the Neck

As discussed previously, the best treatment for arthritis is exercise and stretching. Muscles that are strong and flexible can overcome the rust of arthritis and its pain. One of the areas of the body that is prone to the development of arthritis and disc degeneration is the neck. While we may exercise muscles for other parts of the body, we rarely exercise our neck muscles.

Many of us will try to perform range-of-motion type exercises while we are sitting or standing. This does not tend to provide sufficient exercise for the neck muscles. Because the head sits nicely balanced on top of the spine, moving the neck through its various ranges of motion doesn't require a lot of muscle effort. Holding the head at the end of its range of motion, however, does require effort on the part of the muscles that have to check further motion. For instance, if you tilt your head forward, the effort by the muscles at the front of the spine (rectus capitus anterior) to actually move the head forward is minimal. However, to hold the neck bent forward for any length of time requires ongoing activation of the muscles at the back of the neck, particularly the trapezius.

Another form of movement many of my patients perform is attempts to crack their own neck. They believe that since the chiropractor or osteopathic physician has cracked their neck, doing so on their own will somehow release restrictions. The truth is that while such self "correction" might produce transient relief from pain and the feeling of restriction, for the most part the relief is only temporary. Worse, if it is performed frequently, there is the tendency for the neck to become hyper-mobile. That is, it becomes difficult for the bones and soft tissues of the neck to hold a normal balanced orientation.

Similarly, many people attempt to relieve discomfort in their neck by rotating the neck through its range of motion. Supposedly this produces a stretching of the various muscles and therefore should increase the range of motion. Often people move their neck through what might be termed the "great circle" starting with bending to one side then rolling the head and neck forward into flexion and then into bending to the opposite side and finally into extension (sky gazing) and back to the initial side bending.

I recall not too long ago a 38-year-old male came into my office with a stiff neck. He could not recall any injury or event that caused his neck to become stiff. He was well-muscled and quite physically active in both his work and play. In the absence of any obvious cause, I treated his neck with osteopathic manipulative treatment to reduce his pain and restore his range of motion. Having done so, I questioned him about what kind of neck exercises or stretches he normally used. He proceeded to demonstrate the Great Circle move. He said he performed this maneuver several times a day. Over the years I have had many patients demonstrate this move as their normal method of loosening their neck.

Unfortunately, the Great Circle move can produce a restriction in one or more of the neck vertebral bones, as it did in George's case. When this happens, the patient may experience a jab of pain or more frequently will notice that the next time they try to turn their neck in a particular direction they can't do it as well and they experience pain.

There are probably a couple of reasons for this self-created restriction. First, the Great Circle maneuver is typically performed in one direction only (most frequently clockwise looking down from above). This produces uneven utilization of the neck muscles and over time can produce fixed patterns of activation and may also differentially strengthen some muscles and cause others to weaken.

Another factor in producing restriction and pain in the Great Circle maneuver may have to do with the anatomy of the neck bones (cervical vertebrae). Recall that each vertebra consists of a body and the posterior boney ring that surrounds and protects the spinal cord. Each cervical vertebra has eight boney projections involved in sliding joints. Because of how these joints are aligned, movements on the diagonal are more likely to end up producing a bind at one or more of the facet joints. When these joints bind, they will cause a decrease in the range of motion between the vertebrae and can cause pain. The Great Circle maneuver involves mostly diagonal movements. Therefore, it can easily produce facet binding and the resulting pain and restriction to the neck.

FOUR QUADRANT NECK EXERCISES

What kind of exercises do I recommend for those who have neck pain and arthritis? This basic set of exercises seems quite easy on the face of it. However, as suggested earlier, a fair amount of the pain we experience in the neck is due to a weakening and atrophy of the muscles that manage the neck particularly when we are erect. The exercises I teach come from a series of old osteopathic strengthening maneuvers taught early in the 20th century. I have not seen them discussed elsewhere. They do seem particularly effective in my patients, even those whose arthritis and pains have reduced their neck to only a few degrees of motion, as was discussed in the case of the patient in the last chapter. The series is named the "Four Quadrant Neck Exercises."

The Four Quadrant Neck Exercises are performed in bed. It doesn't seem to matter whether they are done first thing in the morning or before bedtime at night. The exercise takes only a few minutes. The head, which weighs about eight pounds, is enough weight by itself. Ultimately of course the head is the weight that our neck muscles have to deal with whenever we are erect.

The target is to be able to do 20 of each of four movements. Many of my patients have been shocked by how few they can actually perform the first time they try the movements. They find some movements harder to do and some easier. Do not be upset or ashamed if you can only do one or two repetitions of specific movements. Several things limit people from doing more: pain, weakness, and muscle fatigue. It is only a sign that these muscles are weak and need this type of exercise. The "Four Quadrant Exercises" need to be performed daily. As a number of my patients of many years can attest, these exercises are surprisingly effective.

The Four Quadrant Neck Exercises are performed in bed lying down. The only weight needed is the weight of your head (about 7 or 8 pounds):

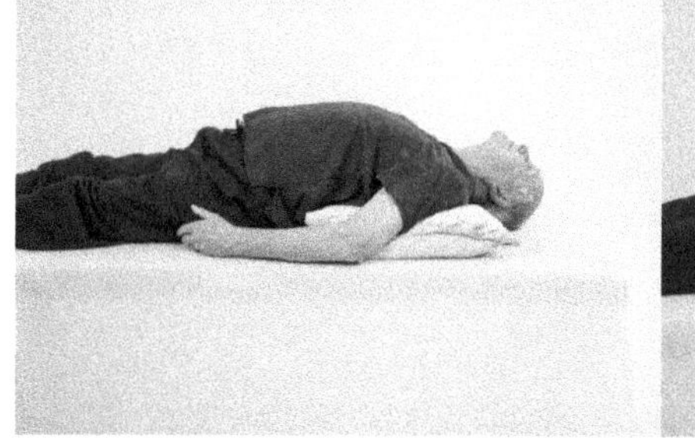 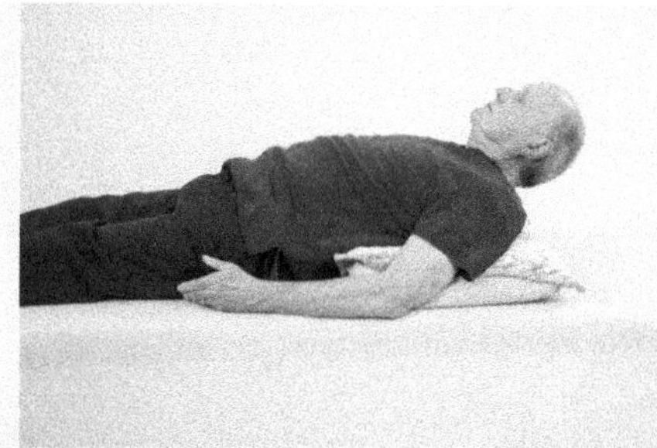

1. Start on your back with a pillow under your shoulders. Alternatively, you can start with your shoulders at the edge of the bed and your head and neck hanging off the bed. In either case allow your head to extend backwards (Fig. 16-1a).
2. From this position, bring your head up and your chin toward your chest Fig. 16-1b). This uses the muscles on the front side of the neck.
3. Now allow your head and neck to return to the extended position.
4. You want to perform as many neck flexion moves as you can, up to a total of 20. Do not be alarmed if you can only do a few flexions at first. This is merely a sign that muscles on the front of your neck were weaker than you realized.

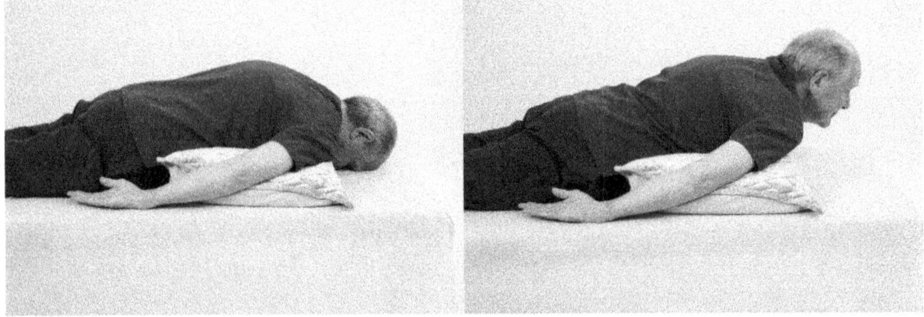

5. Next turn over on your stomach. Again, there should be a pillow under your chest and your head should rest on the bed (Fig. 16-1c).
6. Let your head and neck go forward by relaxing. From this flexed neck position, you will lift your head up, extending it toward your back (Fig. 16-1d). This exercises the muscles at the back of the neck.
7. Now allow it to return to the flexed position. Again, do as many as you can, up to 20.

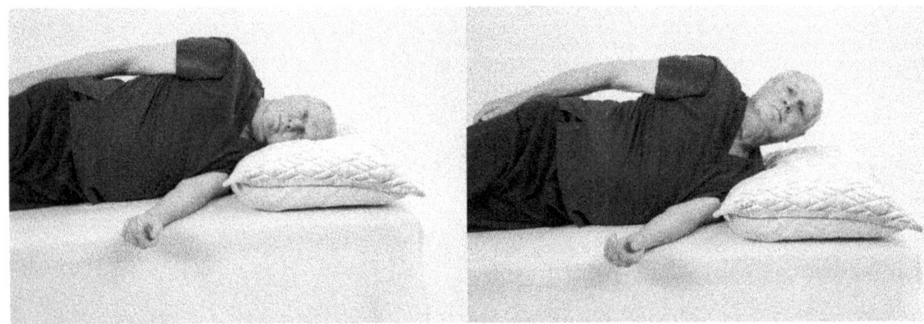

8. Now roll up onto your left side. Allow your neck to relax toward the bed or floor. You may need to rest your head on a pillow initially (Fig. 16-1e).
9. Using the muscles on the upper side of the neck, pick your head up trying to bend the head and neck toward the side of your upper or right shoulder (Fig.16-1f). Again, the target is to be able to do 20 of these side-to-side movements.
10. Finally roll onto your right side and again do side-to-side motions toward the upper or left shoulder. Once again, your target is to be able to do 20 of these side-to-side motions.

It may require several months of daily Four Quadrant Neck Exercises before you are able to do 20 of each of the four exercises. Eventually you will find you can do 20 of each move easily and efficiently. Most likely there will be a major decrease in neck pain. I would recommend that you continue to do these exercises daily or at least four days a week for the rest of your life if you have significant arthritis of the neck. You will definitely see the benefit in decreased neck pain and increased mobility.

NECK POSTURE

As discussed in the chapter on posture, the neck is frequently subject to pain and restriction of motion due to abnormal posture. Whether this stems from inactivation of neck muscles due to trauma or from mere postural decompensation, the results are the same. Remember that people with this kind of neck problem tend to stand with their neck and head held forward. There is an accentuation of the transition curve between the forward arch of the upper back and the backward arch of the neck, producing almost an S-shape. They have rounded shoulders and may be developing what was historically termed a "dowager's hump." Often, they have pain mostly at the base of the neck, but also at the base of the skull. Typical exercises to straighten their posture have involved strengthening the trapezius muscles and sometimes the levator scapulae muscles, assuming that these are weak. However, no amount of exercise seems to correct the problem.

When Dr. Vleeming introduced the idea that certain posture muscles can drop out of their normal use patterns causing chronic low back pain (see Chapter 12), I began to suspect that similar events might be involved in some types of chronic neck pain and postural decompensation. In particular I have found that those with pain at the base of the neck and an S-shape cervical thoracic junction tend not to use some deep muscles that bridge between the back of the neck and the upper thoracic spine. These muscles are called the posterior scalenes. The primary action of these muscles seems to be that of flattening this S-shape. When the posterior scalenes are active they allow an erect posture for the head, neck and upper back. It appears that many of those with the increased S posture in this area have inactivated posterior scalene muscles. One way to reactivate these muscles is to perform a direct feedback exercise that seems to recapture the normal postural use of the muscles when you are erect. I will warn you that these exercises are not entirely comfortable and can produce some pain from the muscles during the period when they are transitioning from inactive to being tonically active while you are erect.

The feedback reactivation exercise for the posterior scalene is similar to the "Head Nods from the Front" exercise discussed above.

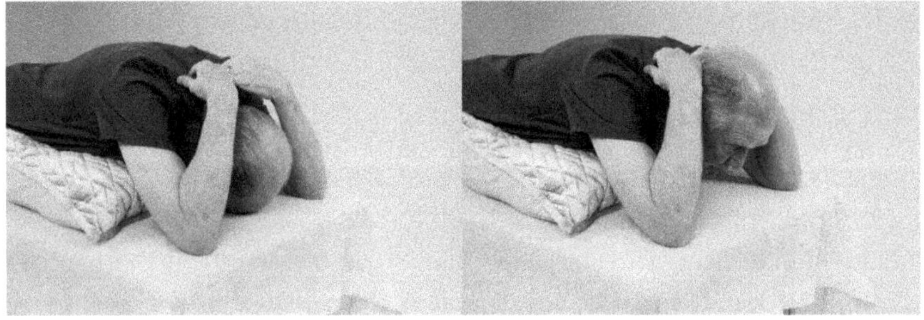

1. Start face down on your tummy on the bed or any supportive surface. Put a pillow under your chest or just lie flat on the bed on your tummy. Place your hands on your shoulders at the base of the neck. Use your fingers to press firmly on both sides of the spine just below the prominence where the neck joins the upper back (Fig. 16-2a).
2. Lift your head off the bed, bending your neck backwards (Fig. 16-2b). It is OK to hold the neck in the extended position for a few seconds.
3. The target is 5 to 10 backward extensions once a day.

My experience with these feedback exercises is that the accented head forward posture begins to resolve almost the first time this exercise is done. However just as the postural decompensation took a long time to develop, it will take a long time for the changes to become permanent. You will need to do this exercise every day for at least six months, and several times a week thereafter, to keep the body aware of and using these posterior scalene muscles.

Recall that the other component in neck posture changes is the relationship between the neck and the mechanics of the shoulders and arms. When we sit with our hands palm down on our legs, the shoulders are rolled forward and inward. In this position it is easy to bend the head down and forward. As I discussed in the chapter on posture, I cannot emphasize strongly enough the need to sit with our hand palms facing upward. This rotates our shoulders outward and backward. The palms-up position naturally keeps the head aligned with the sacrum. When standing or walking we need to avoid having our arms at our sides with the palms facing backward. We do not need to stand or walk with our palms facing forward which is very awkward. The military stance with our palms facing our legs and thumbs forward is sufficient. We need to remember that sitting with our palms face down on our legs and walking with our palms facing backward are cultural norms, so we need to be vigilant to prevent reverting to hand and arm positions that encourage the head thrust forward position.

CHAPTER 17
The Limbs

One of the most interesting facts about the musculoskeletal system is that there are 26 bones in each hand and 25 in each foot. Together the feet and hands amount to 102 bones. Additionally, the arm and shoulder contain five more bones and each leg three bones. Considering the fact that there are only 206 bones in the body, the legs and arms account for more than 50 percent of all the bones in the body.

In most people the arms and legs are mostly muscle and bone by weight and volume. The two legs of the average person are together about 40 percent of the total body weight. Medicine, in general, may give our limbs little focus. However, as the primary instruments allowing us to move around in and manipulate the space around us, they are incredibly important.

THE HAND

Our hands are superbly sensitive and flexible instruments that allow us to skillfully interact with the world and its objects. We can write, paint, feed ourselves, play musical instruments, massage and manipulate other bodies, build buildings, build and operate machines, operate on bodies including eyes and brains and literally thousands of other operations in our world all because of the wonderful dexterity and sensitivity of our hands.

We take our hands for granted ... until we can no longer do so because of damage or disease. Each of the bones of the wrist interact with each other and the long bones of the forearm and provide the base on which the thumb and fingers operate. Many of the hand bones have joints with three or four other bones. Each joint must move smoothly and the bones must retain proper alignment with each other. If they go out of alignment, such as happens when we fall and catch ourselves with the palms of our hands, there will be restriction of motion in the wrist, our grip strength will be diminished and typically there will be pain when we use that hand.

Similarly, if one of the nerves to the hand is damaged, we can lose strength, sensation and dexterity. The nerves can be damaged by compression or actual tearing or even by change in their metabolic environment such as occurs with diabetes. Injury in our neck vertebrae, compression of the nerves at our shoulder, elbow or even at the wrist can lead to a decline or even loss of hand function.

Arthritic changes in the joints of the hand can lead to loss of strength and ability to use the hand. This is especially true in rheumatoid arthritis where the fingers deviate away from the thumb and can no longer be used to grip things or perform normal independent movement of the fingers. In advanced osteoarthritis the finger joints may become enlarged and frozen.

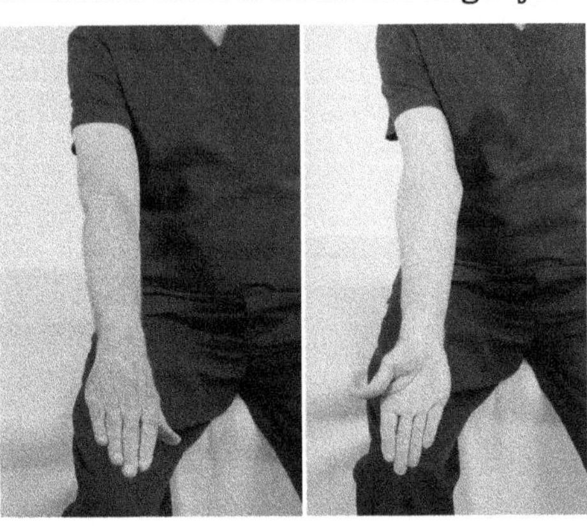

THE ELBOW

The elbow is a complex structure involving joints between three bones: the radius and ulna in the forearm and the humerus of the upper arm. In chapter 2 we discussed a movement unit involving two opponent muscles providing flexion and extension across a joint. The example shown in Figure 2-5 is the elbow. The upper muscle, the biceps, produces elbow flexion and the lower muscle, the triceps, causes elbow extension. Although both muscles actually cross two joints, the elbow and the shoulder, they play only minor roles in shoulder movement. The elbow joint is also structured to allow the forearm to rotate along its long axis, approximately 180 degrees (Fig. 17-1a, b).

The muscles that move the wrist, fingers and thumb are mostly in the forearm and their tendons attach at the elbow. Those that straighten the fingers out and lift the wrist (extension) attach to the outer part of the elbow known as the lateral condyle. The muscles that bend the fingers and thumb and flex the wrist attach to the medial side of the elbow, the medial condyle.

Occasionally we will see restrictions in the head of the radius at the elbow that will keep the forearm from rotating along its long axis. The radial head is part of the complex at the lateral condyle of the elbow. Most of the time, pain and limitation of radial head motion occurs because of restrictions of the wrist. Correction of the wrist restriction allows restoration of forearm rotation.

THE SHOULDER

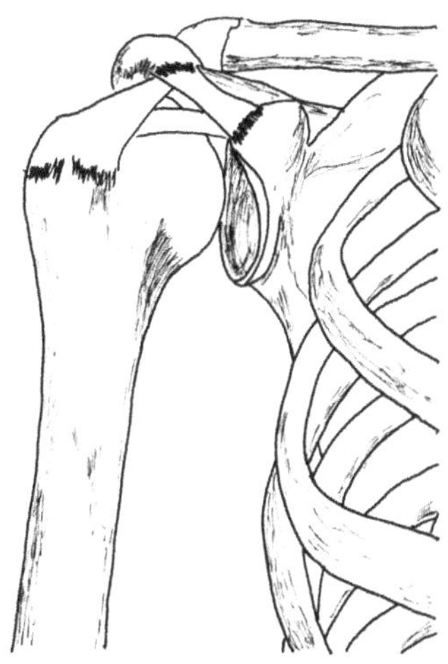

It has been said that the human shoulder is one of the most complex joints in the body. The arm attaches to the body through joints at either end of the collarbone (clavicle). It is worth emphasizing that the only joints attaching the arm and shoulder to the rest of the body are between the collarbone and the middle front chest wall, the sternum. All other attachments are muscles and tendons. The shoulder itself is made up of three bones: the scapula, commonly termed the wing bone, the collarbone (clavicle), and the humerus (the long bone of the upper arm). The scapula and clavicle form a cage around the upper part of the joint, keeping the ball at the upper end of the humerus from moving upward. The bony receiving cup is part of the scapula (Fig. 17-2). It is about the size of a quarter and very shallow. The figure shows a gap in the joint. In the living shoulder the ball would be right next to the receiving cup. To wrap around the humerus ball and give it a more cup-like receiving surface there is a large fibro-cartilage rim (the labrum) that extends up from the small boney receiving surface.

ROTATOR CUFF

The rotator cuff of the shoulder is not really what it sounds like. It is the tendons of four muscles. Each muscle attaches to the shoulder blade. The tendon of each muscle attaches to the bone of the upper arm, the humerus. Each muscle contributes to the possible movement of the arm at the shoulder. Together they also cage the ball of the humerus, holding it in its socket. Together the bone and rotator cuff structures make up a flexible joint that has more than 180 degrees of movement front to back, 160 degrees side to side, and more than 90 degrees movement up and down to the side.

Three of the rotator cuff muscles are responsible for rotating the humerus along its long axis. The fourth rotator cuff muscle works with the cap muscle of the shoulder (the deltoid) to lift the arm to the side. All of the rotator cuff muscles attach to the scapula with very short and broad tendons. Figure 17-2 shows the supraspinatus tendon, one part of the rotator cuff, attaching to the top of the ball of the humerus. Their other ends attach near the head of the humerus. Typically, the rotator cuff muscles and tendons are tough and strong for their size but do not bulk up with exercise the way other muscles of the shoulder can.

When any of the rotator cuff tendons tear or fray, the structural integrity of the shoulder is compromised. Injury to one or more of the rotator cuff tendons also decreases the ability of the shoulder to move and lessens its strength. One or more of the normal motions of the shoulder will be limited. The most common event is to have a partial tear of the tendon of the muscle, supraspinatus, that helps lift the arm to the side.

If there is a partial tear of one or more of the rotator cuff muscles, you will feel pain as you try to move the shoulder. The pain feels like it is inside the shoulder but may be hard to isolate. Although partial rotator cuff tears are fairly common, doctors and physical therapists are quick to conclude that a tear is responsible for shoulder pain. A proper diagnosis involves assessing weakness and pain with specific motions. Otherwise only an MRI will provide an accurate diagnosis.

Generally, the treatment for a partial rotator cuff tear is conservative. Rest with no motion under stress or weight for three to six weeks. Continuing range of motion exercises are reasonable during this initial period as the body builds scar tissue in the area of the tear. After about six weeks exercises involving progressively increasing weights or elastic bands will help the scar tissue to remodel into tissue that can handle normal use of the muscle and tendon.

If all of the rotator cuff tendons tear, the shoulder is limited in its movement and very unstable. It is almost impossible to move such a damaged shoulder. This will probably require surgery and a long rehabilitation.

OTHER SHOULDER MUSCLES

There are a number of other muscles that cross the shoulder joint and contribute to its motion. As mentioned in discussing the elbow, both the triceps and biceps cross the shoulder joint. Others include the pectoral muscles which pull the arm down and forward and teres major, which helps pull the arm down when it has been lifted to the side.

Finally, there are a series of muscles that attach to the scapula. These include the rhomboids, attaching to the posterior chest and spine, levator scapula, attaching to the neck, latissimus dorsi, attaching to the lower back and serratus, attaching to the lateral chest wall below the armpit (axilla).

Two of these muscles can become significant sources of pain. The levator scapula normally acts to stabilize the shoulder blade as you move the arm at the shoulder. The levator scapula muscles are frequently a source of pain when the head and neck are bent down and forward for prolonged periods because they are acting as brakes to prevent the head from falling down onto the chest.

On some occasions the biceps muscle at the shoulder also can become a severe problem. The biceps is responsible for bending the elbow. Biceps means "two heads" in Latin. It is named this because it has two separate tendons at the shoulder. One, termed the short head, attaches to the front of the scapula just below the joint between the scapula and the collarbone. The other tendon runs in a groove on the front surface of the head (ball) of the humerus before attaching to another part of the scapula. This second tendon is termed the long head or bicipital tendon. As long as the bicipital tendon stays in its groove the biceps work well and comfortably as we bend the elbow.

However, there are movements that potentially can dislodge the long head of the biceps from its groove. In the worst-case scenario, the person reaches down behind the body with the arm and picks up something that has some weight like a bag of groceries or a briefcase. If they simultaneously lift the load up and over the shoulder and then bring it to the front of the body with the elbow partially bent, the bicipital tendon may bowstring, popping laterally out of the groove. Pain may not be felt immediately, but within a day or two it can become quite severe and burning. It spreads across the front of the shoulder and down the arm. The pain is frequently nauseating and is bad enough that the normal response is to stop using the shoulder. Unfortunately, the only answer is to find someone who knows how to diagnose and reduce this tendon dislocation. In the more common, relatively minor case, the tendon may slip medially. The pain may be less, but no less bothersome. In both cases prolonged use of the arm in spite of the tendon dislocation will tend to over-stretch the tendon.

PAIN AND THE SHOULDER

Probably because of the intensity of use of the shoulder and because its structure is much less robust than those of the hips and knees, the shoulder has a high number of pain nerves. Presumably this large representation of pain nerves prevents us from using the shoulder inappropriately and possibly causing injury. What this means is that tears to the rotator cuff and fractures of any of the bones of the shoulder cause a lot of pain. Remember as well that pain from the left shoulder can be mistaken for pain from the heart or esophagus because the pain nerves are shared.

THE HIP

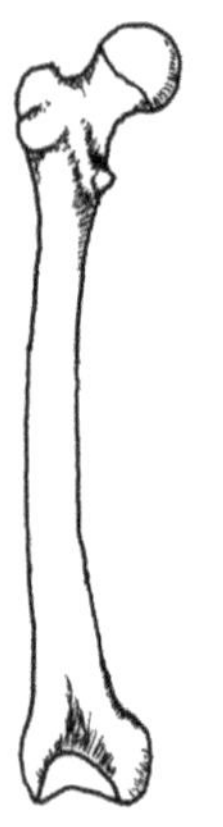

What we commonly refer to as the hip is a mixture of the buttock muscles discussed in the Pelvis chapter, the joint between the innominate bone and the thigh bone (femur) and the area where the thigh bone bends to become the long bone of the thigh. The actual hip joint is behind the area commonly referred to as the groin. If one looks at the thigh bone from the front, it has the same basic shape as a hockey stick (Fig. 17-3a). The ball is on the short arm of the hockey stick and makes a joint with the innominate bone. The outside of the thigh bone where it makes its bend is termed the greater trochanter. The greater trochanter is where the four buttock muscles and part of the IT band attach.

The hip joint is prone to developing osteoarthritis particularly in those who are older or overweight or both. It can be announced by increased stiffness and sometimes pain in the hip when the movement is larger than that required by walking. Often the development has been too subtle to notice until the arthritis is quite advanced. At present there is very little we can do to arrest the development of hip joint osteoarthritis. Working on strengthening muscles and stretching their tendons to maintain flexibility can ward off the severe pain and restriction that can occur when the joint reaches the bone-on-bone stage. At this time the only treatment for end-stage osteoarthritis of the hip is surgical replacement of the joint.

HIP BURSITIS

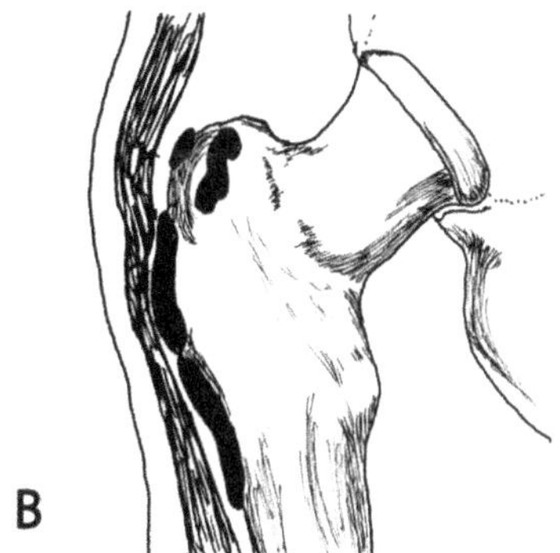

Recall that a bursa is a flattened sack that extends from joints so that it lies under tendons to protect them from rubbing on each other and on the bone. In the hip the major bursa is about 4 to 5 inches away from the actual joint. The hip bursa is on the outside of the thigh bone (femur) at the trochanter (shown in black on Fig. 17-3b). The trochanter bursa lays under buttock muscle tendons just before they attach to the trochanter. Inflammation in the trochanter bursa seems to occur spontaneously. It can occur at any age (the youngest patient with trochanter bursitis in my practice was 14 years old, the oldest was 106). Generally, it occurs without an identifiable cause (termed idiopathic) although it is more common among those over the age of 50. Sometimes, if we fall on the outside of the hip, bruising will occur inside the bursa, causing a traumatic bursitis. Bursitis of the hip can last as long as 18 months before it resolves.

The primary symptoms of hip bursitis are pain in the gluteal muscles and along the IT band, including specifically when one lies on that hip in bed. Exercise does not typically cause the pain to get worse. Because of the protective reflexes the hip is generally up-slipped or sheared upwards on the side of the bursitis, producing what appears to be a shortened leg. The only generally successful treatment of trochanter bursitis of the hip is to inject the bursa with a steroid.

ILIOTIBIAL BAND

We already discussed the iliotibial band or IT band when we discussed the pelvis. Because it is a major structure of the thigh, a few facts bear repeating. The IT band is a specialized tendon that is found on the lateral or outside surface of the thigh. It is the thickest and largest tendon in the body. Frequently it is described as a ligament. However, it does have a muscle body, called the tensor fascia lata, that attaches to the pelvis. The tensor fascia lata is relatively small and basically acts as a tensioner for the IT band. The IT band acts as a brake to keep the leg from going too far toward the opposite side of the body. It is a stabilizer helping to keep the leg from collapsing inward when we stand and walk. The IT band starts at the outside boney crest of the pelvis and attaches both to the long bone of the thigh (femur) and to the bones below the knee.

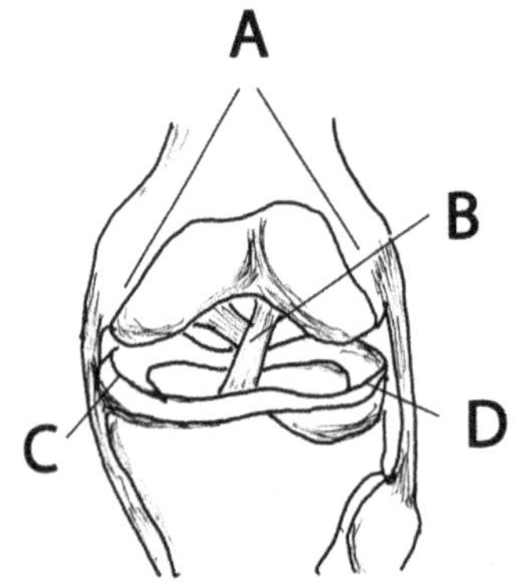

THE KNEE

The knee is one of the primary weight-bearing joints of the body. The lower end of the femur has two rounded knobs that sit on a more-or-less flat plate formed by the top end of the tibia, the primary long bone of the lower leg. The knobs of the femur, termed condyles, are much wider than the long bone itself (Fig. 17-4a). In between the two condyles are two internal ligaments called the cruciates (Fig. 17-4b). As discussed earlier, they act to limit how much the condyles can glide front to back. They also help prevent the knee from hyperextending. On the medial or inside surface of the tibial plateau is a half-moon shaped fibro-cartilage that is higher toward the outside of the joint (Fig. 17-4c). This is the medial meniscus. A similar structure is seen on the lateral surface of the tibial plateau, the lateral meniscus (Fig. 17-4d). When people talk of torn cartilage in the knee, one of these meniscus structures is what has been torn. The function of the meniscus is to change the flat surface of the tibial plateau to a more cup-shaped structure. This allows the knee to flex and extend to a straight line and rotate a little along the line of the long bones without sliding off in a medial or lateral direction. Contributing to the stability of the knee are medial and lateral ligaments, the IT band, as

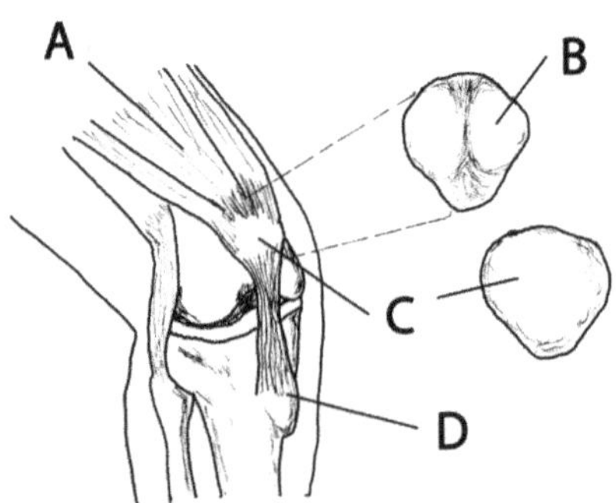

previously discussed, and the muscles that cross the knee.

There are four muscle groups that cross the knee. The first group is the medial thigh muscles (the adductors) that pull the leg in toward the other leg. The second is the hamstrings at the back of the thigh that attach to the back of the tibia and cause the knee to flex. The third group is the calf muscles, some of which send tendons to the back of the femur just above the knee. The fourth are the quadriceps at the front of the thigh which cause the knee to straighten (Fig. 17-5a).

The kneecap or patella (Fig. 17-5b, c) that is seen at the front of the knee connects by a thick ligament to the bony knob on the front of the shin-bone (also known as the tibia) (Fig. 17-5d). The four strap muscles on the front of the thigh are called the quadriceps muscle. They all attach to the top of the knee cap. When these muscles are activated, they pull on the knee cap. In turn, the kneecap pulls on the shin bone and the knee straightens out. On the back side of the kneecap is a ridge (Fig. 17-5b) that lines up with the shin and thigh bones. This ridge normally runs centered between the two knobs (condyles) at the lower end of the thigh bone. Straightening the bent knee works smoothly and well as long as the kneecap ridge rides centered between these two knobs.

THE LOWER LEG

The two long bones of the lower leg differ greatly in thickness. The tibia is much larger in diameter than the bone on the outside, the fibula. The tibia is the primary weight-bearing bone. The fibula attaches to the outside of the tibia just below the knee and at the ankle is the outer part of the joint where it is sometimes termed the ankle bone. The muscles of the lower leg include the calf muscles which attach to the foot by the Achilles tendon and muscles that move the toes and lift the foot.

THE ANKLE AND FOOT

Like the wrist and hand, the lower leg and foot are very complex. As stated earlier there are 25 bones in the foot. The lower leg has two more bones. The bottom end of the tibia becomes the medial condyle or malleolus, which we feel as the inner ankle bone. The bottom end of the lateral strut bone, or fibula, forms the outside ankle bone or lateral malleolus. The top bone of the foot is called the talus and fits between the ends of these two bones. Because of the shape of this complex joint the major motion is to allow the front of the foot to be lifted (extended) or to be pushed down (flexed).

Below and behind the talus is the heel bone or calcaneus. The tendons of the calf muscles attach to the calcaneus as the Achilles tendon. When these muscles contract they lift the heel bone pushing the front of the foot down. If we tear the Achilles tendon we may develop a floppy, unstable foot and ankle.

Attaching between the ankle bones and the talus, calcaneus and other bones of the foot are a number of strong ligaments along the inside and outside of the ankle. These ligaments and some of the tendons crossing the same space act to stabilize the ankle and keep it from rolling inward or outward.

In front of the talus and calcaneus are a couple rows of bones similar to those in the hand. In the foot these form an arch that is supported in part by muscles from the front of the lower leg and in part by the thick and strong plantar fascia. The arch acts as a spring when we walk. When one leg is behind the other and the front of the foot is still on the ground but the heel is lifting off, the arch flattens and tenses. This spring action gives an extra push as we push off with the leg that is behind.

CHAPTER 18
Helping the Arms and Legs

HAND PAIN

The most common form of hand pain, in my experience, is a pain in the area where the thumb becomes part of the hand. This area is fleshy and muscular on the palm side of the hand. Lying under these muscles are some of the carpal bones that make up the hand. The area termed the wrist is two long bones of the forearm termed the radius and the ulna. Together they make up a socket that receives two of the carpal bones, the *scaphoid* on the thumb side and the *lunate* on the little finger side of the hand. Together these four bones create a hinge that allows the hand to flex and extend on the forearm.

Sometimes the bones in this first row of carpals, the scaphoid and lunate, become twisted. This limits the ability of the wrist to flex and extend. Worse, pain develops in the thumb and it becomes difficult to move. Typically, one of two scenarios leads to the twisted scaphoid and lunate. In the first, gripping for a long time, such as with a computer mouse or an ill-fitted tennis racquet or golf club, causes the outer parts of the scaphoid and lunate to be rotated toward the center of the palm and each other. It becomes difficult and painful to extend the thumb completely. There is tenderness over the scaphoid and, in some cases, the lunate. Over time it can produce swelling in the wrist and parts of the thumb. Ultimately it can contribute to developing a form of osteoarthritis. Typically, it also causes limitations of the forearm to roll inward or outward.

If there is tenderness over the scaphoid, but the pain is worse when the thumb is brought across the palm to touch the little finger, the scaphoid and lunate may have been strained in a different fashion. They are outwardly rotated. Most frequently this injury occurs when you hit the palm of your hand forcefully, as when you fall but catch yourself on the palms of your hands. Gripping things becomes painful. You can treat yourself for both forms of wrist restriction:

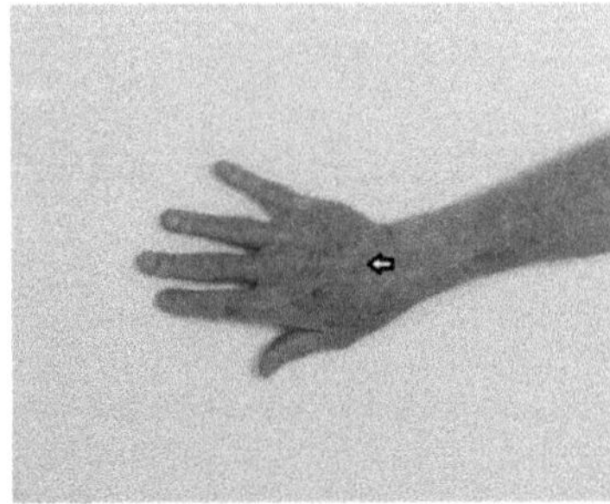

1. On the top surface of the hand locate the high point on the wrist that aligns with the middle finger (Fig. 18-1). If you continue back toward the wrist joint there will be a slight dent. This corresponds to the joint between the scaphoid and the lunate.
2. Place the thumb of your other hand in this dent. There is no need to press firmly.
3. Now bring the thumb and fingers of the hand you are treating together and then spread them apart.
4. Repeat the action of bringing the thumb and fingers together and then spreading them apart five times.
5. Now the thumb and wrist should move more easily without pain.

Recall from Chapter 4 that repetitive compression of the fascia-filled valley formed between the scaphoid and lunate can lead to compression of the nerve and artery that travels through this valley, termed the carpal tunnel. There are a number of scenarios that seem to promote carpal tunnel syndrome. The one reported frequently in the medical literature is jackhammer operators. However, the majority of people who develop carpal tunnel syndrome have never seen a jack hammer. I see it fairly frequently in weightlifters, in tennis players whose racquets are improperly gripped, and golfers who grip their clubs too tightly. I have also seen it in artists who must tightly grip their brush or pencil for long periods when painting fine details. However, one of the most common causes in my practice has been those who spend a lot of time working with a computer mouse while gripping tightly.

The general medical treatment of carpal tunnel syndrome is to inject the carpal tunnel with steroids. By blocking the inflammation and tissue swelling it is hoped that the compression on the nerve will be relieved. A second strategy relies on the idea that during sleep many of those with carpal tunnel syndrome tend to close their hands in a fist and flex the wrist. Wearing a cockup splint that forces the hand to be open and the wrist to be extended will sometimes help relieve the chronic compression of the nerve and artery in the carpal tunnel. Finally, if these two strategies fail, the general recommendation is to perform a surgical release of the tissues. Performing the surgery arthroscopically has a fairly good chance of success, but the definitive surgical release is one that slices through the skin over the carpal tunnel and surgically releases the tightly bound connective tissues in the wrist.

For those who wish to try self-release of their carpal tunnel the first step is to utilize the same treatment used for a wrist restriction discussed above. The second works more directly to stretch the connective tissues within the carpal tunnel.

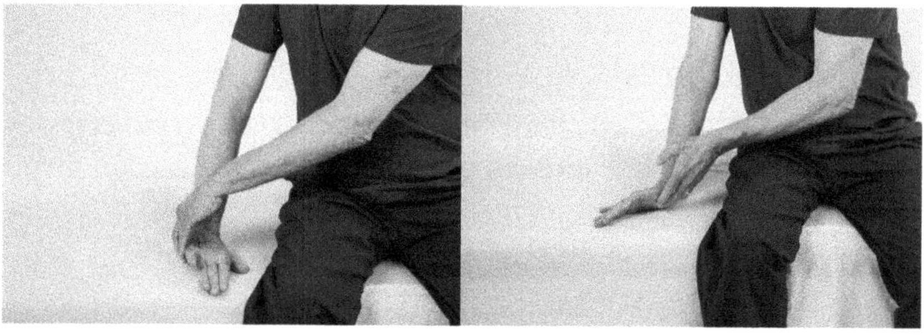

1. Place the hand with carpal tunnel syndrome palm down on a firm surface.
2. Insert fingers from your other hand under the fleshy prominence on the outside of the hand to be treated (the little finger side of the hand) (Fig. 18-2a).
3. Pressing the carpal tunnel hand down, pry up the outside of the hand with your fingers 4-8 times.
4. Now move your fingers so that the tips are under the fleshy part of the palm nearest the thumb (Fig. 18-2b).
5. Again, lift the fleshy prominence 4-8 times.

If you perform this exercise at least once a day you may be able to avoid the medical and surgical treatments. I have also found it useful to use a weightlifter's glove with a palm pad to help protect the carpal tunnel from repetitive pressures.

ELBOW PAIN

Recall that the most common form of pain in the elbow comes from what is commonly termed "tennis elbow." The pain is on the outside of the elbow. It is made worse any time you try to use the hand or wrist. Most of the time tennis elbow develops from repetitive torquing of the wrist.

Not using the affected hand and arm is rarely an option. Ice and heat to the outside of the elbow may help some. Many resort to using a tennis elbow strap. The strap is applied a few inches down the forearm and encircles the forearm. Essentially this strap is compressing the affected muscles, moving the effective tendon insertion down the forearm. This can be effective if used only for the times when extensive use of the hand is necessary. However, you should not wear the strap all the time or the tendons will weaken and become permanently damaged. The typical medical treatment is to inject the tendons with steroids at their insertion on the elbow. While this is sometimes effective, it cannot be repeated without creating the possibility of weakening the tendons.

There are two self-treatments that I recommend for tennis elbow. The first is a way to relax the muscles and their tendons and often provides temporary relief:

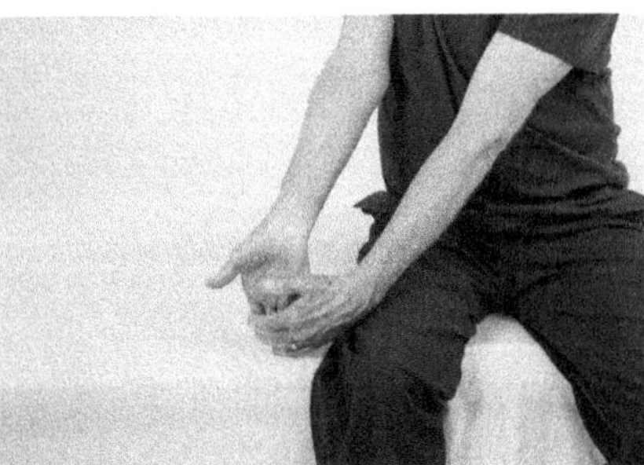

1. Straighten your elbow
2. With the fingers and thumb stretched out, can use your other hand to stretch the fingers and wrist into an extended position (Fig. 18-3). Alternately you can press the hand against a table edge so that the wrist is extended.
3. Hold that position for two minutes.

The second self-treatment is to actually stretch the muscles that attach to the outside of the elbow:

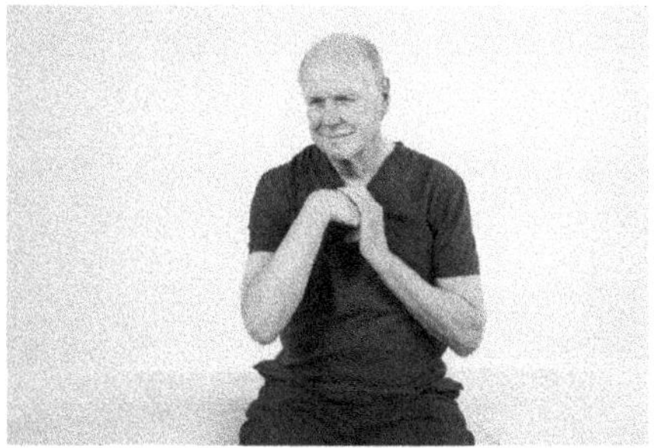

1. Completely bend the elbow so that your hand is in front of your chest.
2. Bend (flex) your wrist and make a fist
3. Wrap your fist with your other hand (Fig. 18-4).
4. Now try to straighten your flexed wrist and extend its fingers with three brief impulses. Don't let the fist, hand and fingers win.
5. Your extensor muscles that attach to the outside of the elbow should be stretched and less tense and painful at the elbow.

SHOULDER RESTRICTIONS

Some of the most common problems in the shoulder stem from inflammation of the muscle tendons. Remember that although the shoulder is a complex joint, it is held together largely by muscles and tendons and the majority of its functional connection with the rest of the body is through muscles. Although the shoulder joints can develop osteoarthritis that can be very limiting, the majority of shoulder pain and dysfunction comes from inflammation. The primary sites of inflammation are the muscle tendons and sometimes in the bursae that protect those tendons from rubbing on each other and on bone.

When any of the tendons develop inflammation, it is termed tendinitis. The most common cause for tendinitis is overuse. This produces pain and inflammation in the tendon and a tendency to avoid using the muscles involved. Remember that not using a muscle and its tendon leads to shortening and eventual muscle atrophy. Paradoxically, the primary treatment for tendinitis is to stretch the muscle. Moist heat and ice can help alleviate any pain involved, but stretching is the cure.

There are a number of bursae that extend from the shoulder joints to positions underlying the shoulder tendons. Although the sure treatment for shoulder bursitis is to inject the bursa with steroid, there is an old osteopathic technique that may allow resolution. This is called the bursa pump. This can be performed actively by you, but sometimes benefits by having someone else perform it on you while you relax. One of the most common sites of bursitis in the shoulder is under the cap muscle at the upper part of the upper arm.

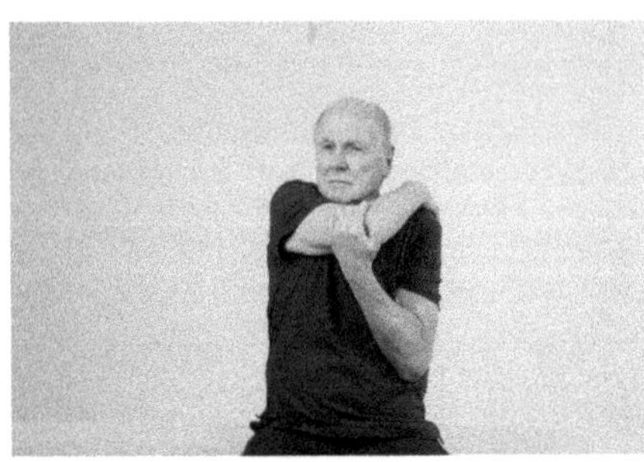

1. Identify a part of the shoulder with pain and swelling. We will assume in this case that it is a bursitis under the deltoid muscle and tendons.
2. Put the muscle and tendons under some tension by bringing the arm forward across the front of the body (Fig. 18-5).
3. Use the other hand to pull the arm with bursitis further across the body.
4. Relax the tension on the arm with bursitis.
5. Repeat the tension/relaxation ten times or more.
6. The repeated tension in the muscle and tendon pushes on the bursa. This pumping action is frequent enough to push the excess fluid out of the bursa and back into the joint where it can be absorbed.

Shoulder injuries and restrictions are fairly common. Minor strains to the joints at either end of the clavicle rarely require treatment since time and activity will generally heal both. However, medical treatment is advised if there is a large joint sprain causing tenderness and a gap greater than 1/3 inch in the joint between the outer end of the clavicle and the scapula (termed the acromio-clavicular joint or AC joint).

Likewise, dislocation of the humerus head in the shoulder joint, while relatively rare, requires immediate medical attention since allowing it to remain dislocated can cause severe pain and inability to use the shoulder. Inevitably the fibro-cartilage rim will be torn. Shoulder dislocation can also compress and damage the blood vessels and nerves to the arm, perhaps permanently.

As discussed in Chapter 4, a frozen shoulder can be prevented by ongoing use and when it does occur can be treated successfully. The primary exercises used to treat a restriction of the shoulder can be used for any situation where a restriction in normal shoulder motion has occurred.

The first two exercise/ stretch methods for the shoulder are both termed "wall walking." The first example is for a restriction in the ability to lift the arm at the shoulder in front. The pectoral muscles are tight preventing the arm from rising. Remember, your arm should be able to go up alongside the ear.

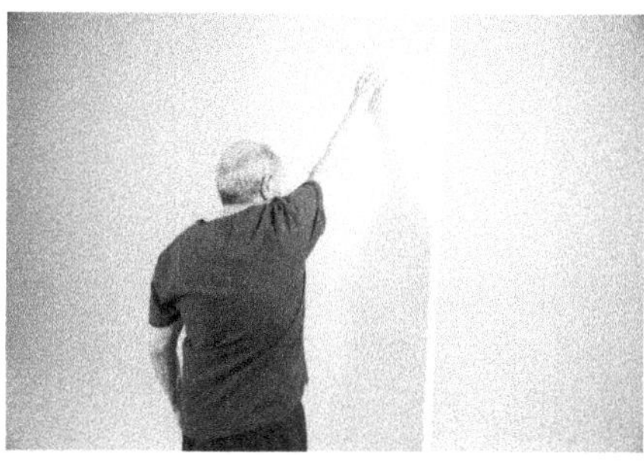

1. Face a wall. Your fingers are partly curved like you are holding a softball. Bring your arm up as high as you can in front. Place your fingers on the wall.
2. Walk with your fingers up the wall like a spider. When you get as high as you can, stop (Fig. 18-6).
3. Briefly (1-2 seconds) and gently try to pull your arm downward without actually moving your fingers on the wall.
4. Repeat the downward push two more times with a pause between each.
5. After the third downward push, walk your fingers up the wall. Surprisingly you will be able to move your arm higher.
6. Repeat the exercise several times a day.

If you have trouble lifting your arm to the side, you can also do "wall walking." Weak deltoid and supraspinatus muscles can limit the ability to raise your arm to the side. However, in a frozen shoulder the limitation is tightness in the muscles used to pull the arm down to your side, latissimus dorsi and teres major. Remember your arm should be able to come up to the side level with the shoulder (90 degrees relative to the body or parallel to the ground).

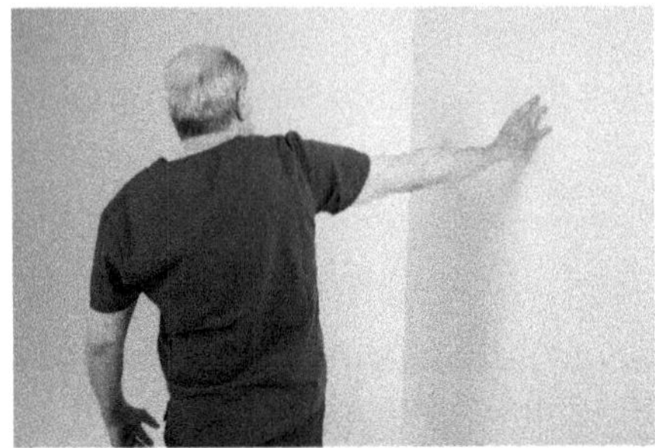

1. Turn so your side is toward the wall. Your fingers are partly curved like you are holding a softball. Bring your arm up as high as you can in front. Place your fingers on the wall.
2. Walk with your fingers up the wall like a spider. When you get as high as you can, stop (Fig. 18-7).
3. Now briefly (1-2 seconds) and gently try to pull your arm downward without actually moving your fingers on the wall.
4. Repeat the downward push two more times with a pause between each.
5. After the third downward push, walk your fingers up the wall. Surprisingly you will be able to move your arm higher.
6. Repeat the exercise several times a day.

If you have a problem bringing your arm across your chest at shoulder level the tightness or stiffness is probably in your rhomboid muscles which are the major muscles on the back of your shoulder. To treat this, you can do the following exercise/stretch:

1. Stand near a wall.
2. Bring your restricted arm forward at shoulder level as possible.
3. Step sideways to the wall until the full length of the arm is resting on the wall (Fig. 18-8).
4. Press briefly with your arm against the wall without moving your body. Do this three times.
5. After the third press pause briefly then rotate your body toward your arm, stretching your shoulder.

When the triceps muscle on the back of the upper arm is tight and tense it can also limit the ability to bring the upper arm across the chest. A tight triceps may also limit the ability to bend your elbow using the biceps muscle. If you have either of these restrictions in, you can try the following stretch. You should be able to place your wrist on the opposite shoulder and the elbow on your chest.

1. Bring your restricted arm as far as you can across the front of your body.
2. Bend that elbow and place that hand on your chest.
3. Bring your other arm under the restricted arm between its elbow and its shoulder.
4. Now bend the elbow of the non-restricted arm. This will block the restricted arm and hold it in place (Fig. 18-9).
5. Now you can gently push the restricted arm away from your body in three brief pulses. Again, do not let the restricted arm actually move.
6. Now you will find you can bring the restricted arm closer to your body.

One of the most common and troublesome pains in the shoulder is found on the back of the shoulder at the upper corner of the shoulder blade. This is where a stabilizer muscle from the neck attaches to the shoulder. The muscle is called levator scapulae. About the diameter of a thick pen, this muscle is often mildly irritated but simply treated as you move your neck to the other side. However, in some cases it becomes chronically inflamed. You can try to stretch it using the following exercise:

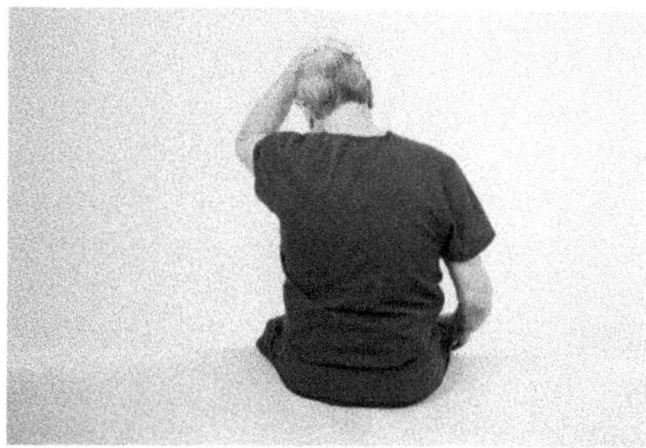

1. Bring your head and neck forward and bend to the opposite side.
2. Using your other arm and hand hold this position (Fig. 18-10).
3. Using your neck muscles, lift your head and neck toward the scapula but not strongly enough to win.
4. Repeat three times.

While these stretching exercises are no substitute for a good diagnostic evaluation, I have had quite a number of patients who have successfully used them without having to go to the doctor. The only limit I would suggest is that if the pain or restriction persists in spite of using these self-treatments, seek medical evaluation and treatment.

Finally, recall from the last chapter the discussion about a possible dislocation of the long head of the biceps tendon from its groove on the head of the humerus. Although this injury is not that common, it is a leading cause of major shoulder pain. Frequently it is confused with the pain from tears of the rotator cuff but it is much more treatable. As stated before, the primary function of the biceps is to bend the elbow. There are two tendons that attach the biceps to the shoulder. The long head or bicipital tendon runs in a groove in the humerus head before attaching to the shoulder near the joint between the collarbone and the shoulder bone. The groove provides a point of leverage that amplifies the strength of the biceps in bending the elbow. There are certain movements that can cause the bicipital tendon to dislocate from its groove. Most involve trying to lift or pull a heavy or resisting object from behind the body. The most common bicipital dislocation is medial to the groove. A bicipital dislocation produces pain focused at the front of the shoulder but it can radiate all over the shoulder and the front of the chest. Using the shoulder is very painful, particularly when it involves bending the elbow. Shoulder pain due to a bicipital dislocation includes point tenderness at the front of the shoulder over the ball of the upper arm. Another clue is that the biceps is sore all the way down to the elbow. If you have a bicipital dislocation, there is a self-treatment that is worth a try.

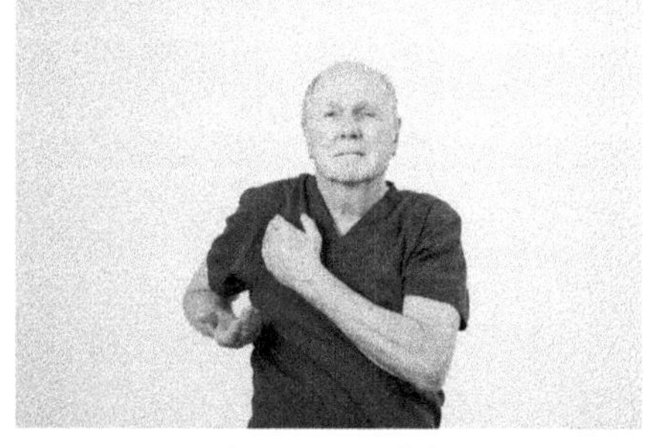

1. Press a finger of the opposite hand on the tenderness on the ball of the shoulder (Fig. 18-11A). You will need to continue pressing on the tender tendon throughout this self-treatment.
2. Bend the elbow of the injured arm as much as possible. Bring the elbow back behind the shoulder. The palm of the hand is facing upward (Fig. 18-11A).

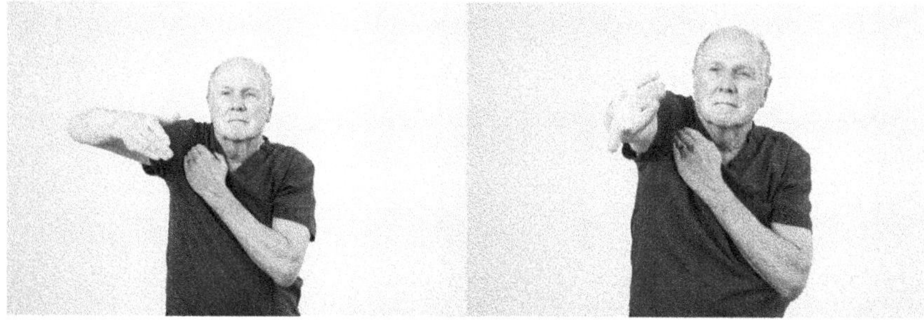

3. Lift the elbow up and begin to swing it forward (Fig. 18-11B). This will feel awkward.
4. Now begin to straighten the elbow out in Front of you. At the same time rotate your hand and wrist to face away from your body (Fig. 18-11C).
5. If you have brought the tendon back into the groove you may feel it during the self-treatment. The tenderness over the tendon will disappear as will your shoulder pain.

In order to tighten the bicipital tendon and hold it in place it is useful to perform biceps hammer curls for a few weeks using a hand weight in the range of 2-5 pounds. To do a hammer curl hold your elbow against your side. Your elbow should start straight or extended. Hold the weight with your wrist and palm facing your side. Now slowly bend your elbow until it is fully flexed. Finally extend the elbow again. That is one repetition. The ideal is to do at least twenty repetitions every day.

HIP PAIN AND BURSITIS

As in the shoulder, pain in the hip and buttocks is most frequently a sign of tension in the muscles and tendinitis. The muscle and tendon will be tender when you push on them. Again, there are two basic methods for resolving tendinitis.

For relaxation, find a leg position where the tenderness and pain goes away. For the buttock muscles this is typically with the hip flexed to about 90 degrees or with the hip flexed at 90 degrees and the leg spread to the side. For the IT band the extended leg is simply spread out to the side. The other methods involve stretching the muscles and their tendons. Stretches for the gluteal muscles and the IT band were discussed and demonstrated in Chapter 14.

When there is swelling and inflammation in the greater trochanter bursa of the hip it is termed a greater trochanter bursitis. Many people are only too happy to have the physician inject the bursa with steroids because the resolution of their pain is rapid. Others would prefer to use more natural means. Recall that this bursitis may last up to 18 months before it spontaneously resolves. It is sometimes worth the effort to use a bursa pump technique to speed recovery.

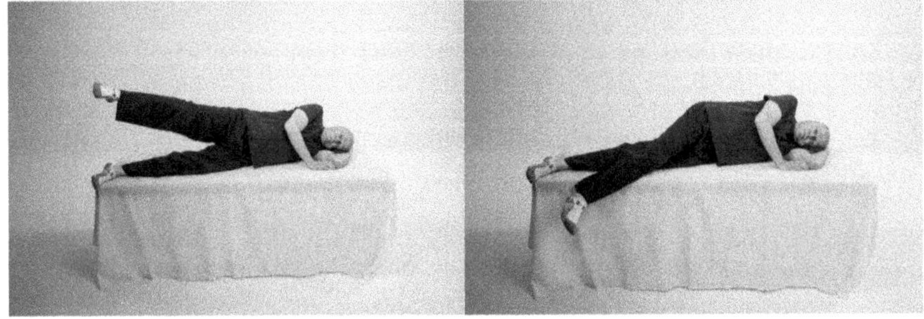

1. Relax the muscles and tendons that attach over the trochanter bursa by shortening. To do this you can lie on your side on a bed or table. The bursitis side is up. Lift the leg up to the side a little (Fig. 18-12A).
2. Now allow the leg to drop forward in front of the other leg (Fig. 18-12b).
3. Bring the leg back into the original position, lifted to the side.
4. Repeat 10 times or more.

An alternative that sometimes works almost as well is performed sitting:

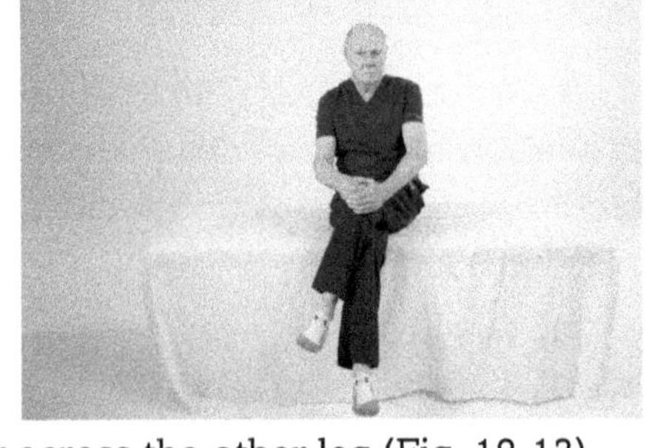

1. Sit on a chair or stool. The thigh of the leg with bursitis rests on top of the other thigh. This position does not allow the tendons to relax.
2. With your hands on the lower thigh of the leg with bursitis push the thigh further across the other leg (Fig. 18-13).
3. Stop pushing. Allow the leg with bursitis to move back to its original position.

4.   Because the motion of pushing on the bursa is more limited it may require being repeated 10 to 20 times and repeated a couple of times a day for several days before improvement is noted.

Both hip bursa pump techniques work by using repeated tension in the muscle and tendons of the buttocks and leg to push on the bursa. Again, this pumping action may be enough to push the excess fluid out of the bursa and back into the joint where it can be absorbed.

KNEE PAIN

Frequently I see patients whose major complaint is knee pain. When they try to ride a bicycle or walk up or down stairs or stand up from sitting in a chair at least one of their knees hurts a lot. Maybe the pain is bad enough they feel like it is impossible to go up and down stairs. More likely they are reduced to climbing up and down stairs one step at a time, first putting one foot on the next step and then the other and pulling themselves along using the railing. They feel like their leg muscles are so weak that they will become unable to walk. They are sure that their knees have developed severe arthritis since there is grating and popping as they walk or even bend their knees. The fear is that they have become so arthritic that their knees will have to be replaced.

When their knee is analyzed, there is no swelling or laxity. There is no evidence of torn cartilage. There may be some joint space narrowing by touch or X-ray but not enough to present as "bone-on-bone." What they do have is grating under the kneecap.

In medical terms the problem is patella-femoral syndrome or, at its worst, chondromalacia patella, which, in fact, is a form of arthritis. However, the problem is not due to arthritis. It is due to an imbalance in the quadriceps muscle that straightens the knee.

As discussed in the last chapter the quadricep muscles attach to the top of the kneecap. There is a tendon that then attaches between the bottom of the kneecap and a projection of bone on the upper fibula. There may be an imbalance in the four muscles of the quadriceps. If the middle two strap muscles are stronger than the lateral two muscles, the kneecap will move inward toward the other leg. If the kneecap moves toward the outside, the lateral strap muscles are stronger.

Remember that the kneecap has a ridge along its back side that runs in the valley formed by the two knobs at the end of the femur. The underside of the kneecap will rub on one of the knobs if the kneecap tracks toward the inside or outside of the knee during straightening. Over time the cartilage on the underside of the kneecap and on the thigh bone knob starts to wear down. This roughening produces popping, grating, and pain whenever the knee is straightened. Frequently a sense of muscle weakness in the thigh starts to develop as well. This is the patellofemoral syndrome or chondromalacia patella.

How do you know if your knee pain is being caused by a miss-tracking kneecap? As suggested above, having popping or grating sounds when straightening your knee is one clue. If you have knee pain, grating or popping when going up or down stairs or getting up from a chair you have a second clue. The feeling that your leg is somehow weak and could give way is also common. Tenderness along the inside and/or outside of the kneecap is another possibility. To really figure this out, sit on something high enough that you can freely swing your knee. Grab your kneecap between your thumb and index finger so you can feel what the kneecap does when you straighten your knee. If the kneecap moves toward the other leg or away from the other leg as you straighten your leg, you have a miss-tracking kneecap. Often you can feel a gap under the kneecap on the side toward which it drifted. What these signs indicate is that there is a muscle imbalance in the quadriceps muscles.

It is surprisingly easy to correct this knee problem and the fix is at least semi-permanent. What we use is an exercise that will rebalance the strength of the four strap muscles that make up the quadriceps. The first example will be for a kneecap that rides toward the other leg (medial mis-tracking).

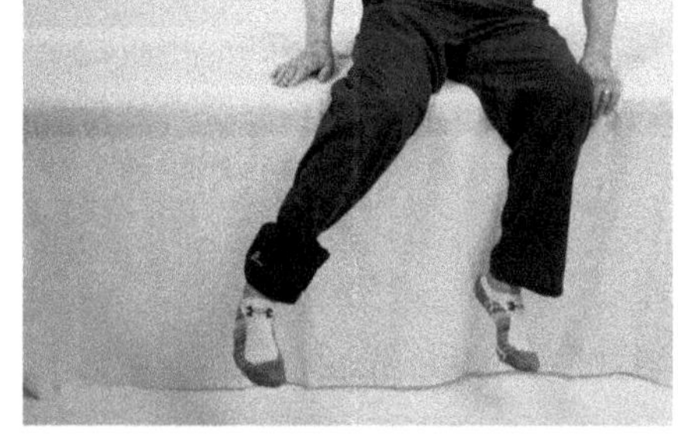

1. Place a one- or two-pound weight around your ankle (150 pennies weighs about a pound; a shoe also generally weighs at least a pound).
2. Sit on a surface high enough so that your feet are off the floor.
3. Roll your thigh inward so your ankle is to the outside of your knee (Fig 18-14a)

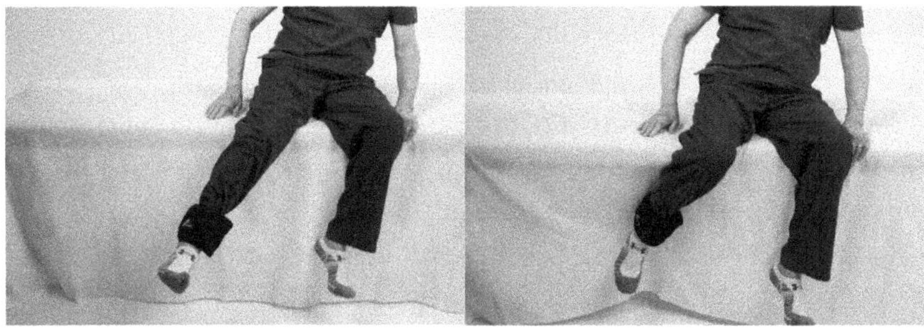

4. Holding this position, swing your foot and lower leg from the back to the front (back and forth) (Fig. 18-14b, c). This activates the outer quadriceps muscles.
5. The target is 50 swings a day for two weeks. After two weeks the quadriceps muscle should be balanced and the kneecap should track properly. As long as it is properly tracking you can stop the exercise. It doesn't matter if a little grating remains.

To treat a kneecap that is tracking towards the outside of the knee (lateral mis-tracking):

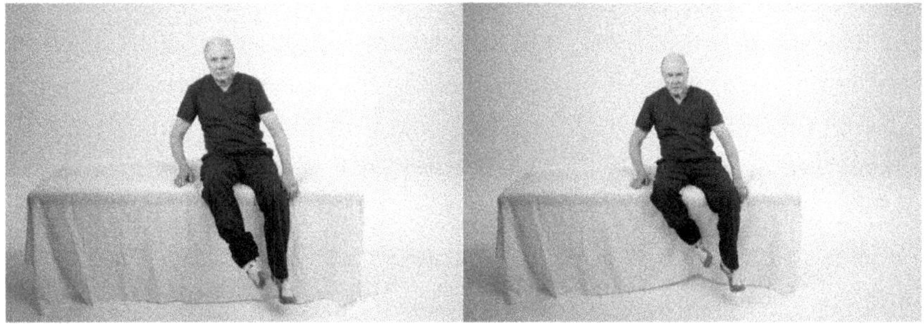

1. Roll the thigh outward so the ankle is closer to the other leg (Fig. 18-15a).
2. Maintain this position while doing 50 front-to-back swings a day for two weeks Fig. 18-15a, b).
3. Do not continue the exercise longer than two weeks or the kneecap may start to swing in the opposite direction.

In more than 20 years of medical practice, this strategy has been successful in dealing with this type of knee pain virtually every time.

ANKLE AND FOOT PAIN

Pain in the feet and ankles is very common. In our culture a lot of it comes from wearing shoes. To understand how this might be we have to look first at how people walk. As very young children when we first start walking, we use our toes a lot, particularly when walking in our bare feet. As the foot that is in back pushes off to bring it to the front the toes actually curl and grip the ground. Older people who walk barefoot continue to curl their toes during the push-off phase of walking. However, those of us who wear shoes most of our walking lives follow what the shoes themselves do: the front part of the shoe and toes bend upward as we push off with the back foot. Over a lifetime the natural tendency to curl the toes during the push-off phase of walking gets lost.

If we look at the foot when it is not weight-bearing, we see that curling the toes down tends to reinforce the natural arch along the bottom of the foot. Lifting the toes up tends to flatten the same arch. Curling our toes requires activating muscles in the lower leg that also help support the arch. A lifetime of not curling the toes leads to weak muscles and loss of arch support. As a result, most of us who reach our middle age are showing signs of loss of the natural foot arch when we stand or walk. This puts considerable strain on the ligaments along the bottom of the foot that also help support the arch. After a while this can result in pain in the foot. Doctors term this pain plantar fasciitis. Other factors that contribute to this painful condition are wearing shoes that are too short and walking all the time in high heels. Both of these tend to cause shortening of the tendons on the top of the foot that pull the toes. Chronic shortening of the great toe tendon often leads the toe bending toward the others, causing a bunion. Chronic shortening of the other toe extensor tendons leads to hammer toes. Both of these conditions reinforce the stretching of the fascia on the bottom of the foot arch, allowing it to flatten.

To treat plantar fasciitis, you need to strengthen the muscles that flex the toes, support the arch and support the ankle. The two recommended exercises are toe scrunches and heel rises.

Toe scrunches:

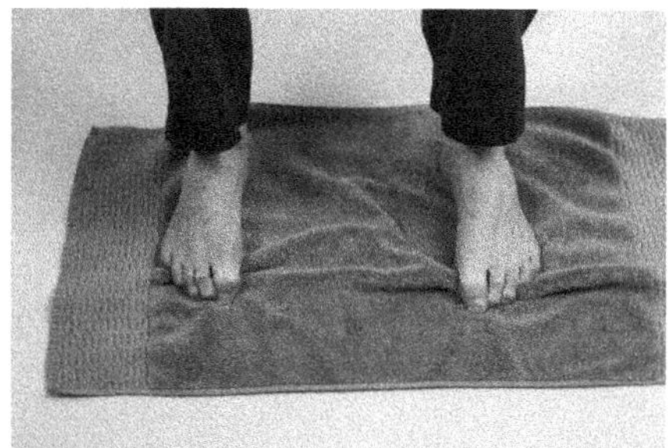

1. Throw a towel on the floor.
2. Make sure your feet are bare.
3. Attempt to grab the towel with both feet by flexing your toes (Fig. 18-16).
4. Do 50 scrunches per day.

Heel rises:

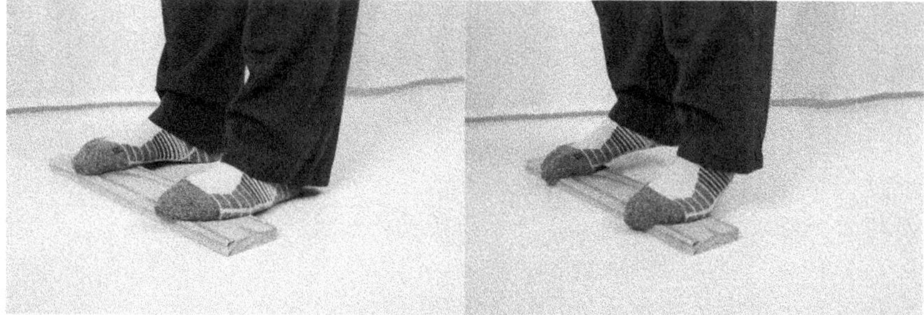

1. Start with a ¾-inch block. A piece of one-by-four works great, although a book or small stack of magazines will also do just fine.
2. In your bare feet, place the balls of both feet and your toes on the block. Your heels are on the floor (Fig. 18-17a).
3. Do heel rises from the block (Fig 18-17b), being sure to touch the heel to the floor with each repetition.
4. When you can do 50 heel rises easily, gradually increase to a 1 ½-inch block (which could be a piece of two-by-four). Remember your heels must drop all the way to the floor.

Heel rises off a block are not the same as doing them off a step. This is true largely because the feet will rarely go into an upwardly flexed position (heel below the forefoot) during the exercise if done off a step. If we actually try to do this off a step, we will tend to fall backwards. The heel rise exercise taught here requires that both feet need to go into both upwardly and downwardly flexed positions in order for this exercise to strengthen the muscles and ligaments to hold the ankles and arches stable. Typically, it takes up to two months for you to notice that your arches are no longer collapsing and the plantar fascia are no longer painful. An additional benefit will be that you will be much less prone to spraining your ankles.

The other common problem with the foot and ankle is a sprain. Typically, this occurs when stepping onto a surface so that the ankle rolls inward or outward. Stepping onto an uneven surface like cobblestone can produce the same result. The tendons and ligaments on the outside or inside of the ankle are overstretched and may develop tears. The amount of stretching and tearing is defined medically as a first-, second- or third-degree sprain. A first-degree sprain is considered mild and is relatively easy to overcome. A third-degree sprain involves complete tearing of major tendons and ligaments and is considered to require surgical treatment. Although the standard medical treatment for first- and second-degree sprains involves the mantra "ace, ice, and elevate," osteopathic physicians have been manipulating the feet and providing early resolution of pain and instability for more than 100 years. Long-term the best thing a person can do after a sprained ankle is to perform the same toe scrunches and heel rises used to treat plantar fasciitis.

CHAPTER 19
Concluding Thoughts

In many ways, this book could be considered a users' guide to our muscles, tendons, ligaments, joints, bones, and nervous system. Most frequently problems in the nerves, central nervous system and muscles and bones announce themselves in the form of pain and restriction. Over the years I have seen many patients who had no idea where to turn when such problems developed in their body. The advice given in this book is not a replacement for a thorough and appropriate diagnosis of your problem. Remember, even though your problem may present as restriction or pain in the muscles, joints and bones, the source may be elsewhere. It is not the intent of this book to present all possible diagnoses or all possible treatments for what appears to be neural, muscle and bone problems. If I have given you a better understanding of what might be going on, then I will have done my job.

Understanding who to turn to is also helpful. In many cases our friends and relatives, and even our doctors, may not know where to turn. Hopefully this book has helped point out some new possibilities in treatment of your problems. In particular since you may not have ready access to a manual medicine or musculoskeletal medicine specialist, stories about some of my patients may help you understand what you are experiencing and point the way to better methods of dealing with your problem. Finally, knowing that there are self-help strategies may make things easier.

Ultimately, as has been pointed out in a number of places, this book should remind you that the upkeep and maintenance of your body is in your hands. Hopefully some of the treatments suggested in this book will be useful additions to your maintenance toolkit.

www.ingramcontent.com/pod-product-compliance
Lightning Source LLC
Chambersburg PA
CBHW052356030726
47599CB00014B/1091